Contents

WEIGHT TRAINING Q&A 2
LEGS 25

Standing Calf Raise......................................26
Bridge 28
Bodyweight Squat..30
Bodyweight Lunge.......................................32
Sumo Squat...34
Stability Ball Hamstring Curl....................36
Step-Up...38
Lateral Lunge 40
Dumbbell Squat..42
Dumbbell Lunge..44
Stability Ball Single-Leg
    Hamstring Curl......................................46
Dumbbell Deadlift......................................48
Split Squat...50
Barbell Deadlift 52
Barbell Squat...54
Dumbbell Straight-Leg Deadlift.............56
Barbell Straight-Leg Deadlift.................58
Barbell Front Squat....................................60

CHEST 63

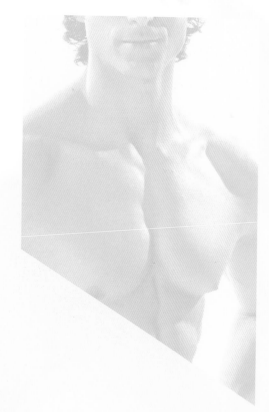

Incline Push-Up...64

Kneeling Push-Up 66

Push-Up..68

Decline Push-Up.......................................70

Dumbbell Chest Press..............................72

Dumbbell Chest Fly 74

Incline Dumbbell Chest Press.................76

Incline Dumbbell Chest Fly 78

Barbell Chest Press....................................80

Incline Barbell Chest Press......................82

Decline Dumbbell Chest Press................84

Decline Barbell Chest Press.....................86

BACK 89

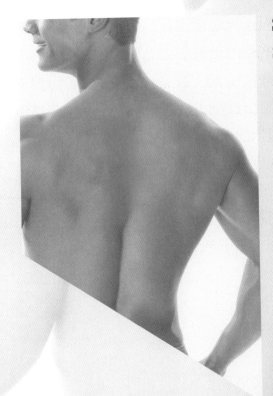

Stability Ball Back Extension 90

Seated Cable Low Row 92

Cable Lat Pulldown................................ 94

Dumbbell T-Bar Row.............................. 96

Dumbbell Pullover 98

Dumbbell One-Arm Row 100

Dumbbell Bent-Over Row 102

Barbell Bent-Over Row 104

Inverted Row....................................... 106

Pull-Up... 108

SHOULDERS 111

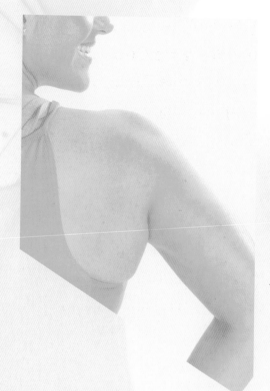

Dumbbell Lateral Raise 112

Dumbbell Front Raise 114

Dumbbell Reverse Fly 116

Dumbbell Upright Row 118

Dumbbell Shoulder Press 120

Cable Lateral Raise 122

Cable Face Pull 124

Barbell Upright Row 126

Barbell Shoulder Press 128

Arnold Press.. 130

ARMS.. 133

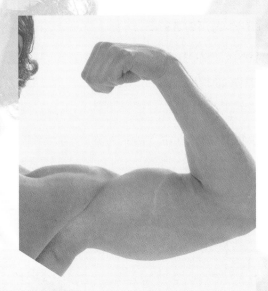

Dumbbell Bicep Curl 134

Dumbbell Bicep Hammer Curl 136

Dumbbell Bicep Reverse Curl 138

Dumbbell Tricep Kickback 140

Cable Bicep Curl 142

Cable Tricep Pushdown 144

Barbell Bicep Curl 146

Barbell Bicep Reverse Curl 148

Bench Dip...150

Barbell Tricep Skull Crusher................152

Bodyweight Dip...154

ABS 157

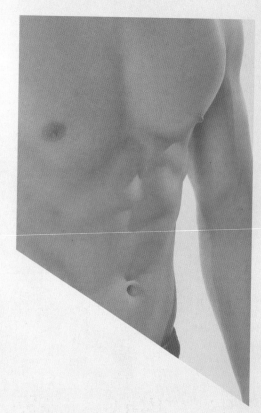

Basic Crunch 158
Stability Ball Crunch 160
Bicycle Crunch 162
Reverse Crunch 164
Cable Crunch Down 166
Sit-Up 168
Wood Chopper 170
Mountain Climber 172
Plank and Side Plank 174
Stability Ball Pike 176
V-Up 178
Hanging Leg Lift 180
Stability Ball Mountain Climber 182

TRENDS 185

MEDICINE BALLS 187
Around the World 188
Worship Stretch 190
Crunch Bounce 192
Ball Slam 194
Push-Up 196
Sit-Up Press 198
Sun God Squat 200
Lunge and Twist 202

BALANCE TRAINERS 205
Wood Chopper 206
Crab Walk 208
Squat 210
Dip 212
Plank 214
Push-Up 216

KETTLEBELLS 219
Figure 8 220
Windmill 222
Swing 224
Reverse Lunge Pass 226
High Plank Row 228
Sit-Up Press 230
Get-Up 232

SUSPENSION BANDS 237
Squat and Single-Leg Squat 238
Chest Press and Chest Fly 240
Row and Reverse Fly 242
Plank and Side Plank 244
Hamstring Roll 246
Bridge 248
Mountain Climber 250

ROUTINES 253

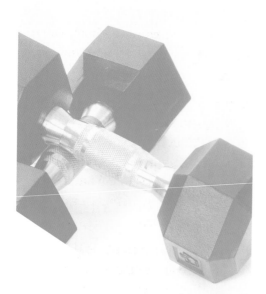

Two-Day Routine 254

Three-Day Routine 257

Four-Day Routine.................................261

Full Body in 15 Routine.........................266

Weight Loss Routine 271

Muscle Gain Routine............................273

Introduction

Embarking on a weight-training routine can feel like a home remodeling project. At first, you're all fired up and eager to get everything started, but after a couple weeks you find yourself anxious and annoyed with how slow the progress is coming.

Don't give up! *Idiot's Guides: Weight Training* covers more than just the basics. In this book, you'll learn the proper technique on how to condition every muscle in your body, when to progress yourself to avoid plateaus, and how to design your own workout routines.

The first six parts in this book contain exercises broken down by muscle groups: legs, chest, back, shoulders, arms, and abs. Each includes fundamental weight-training exercises for that specific group done with free weights or your own bodyweight, organized by difficulty level. The seventh part is devoted to trends, or special equipment used to perform weight-training exercises: medicine balls, balance trainers, kettlebells, and suspension bands. It's important to have a solid foundation with weight-training exercises that use traditional equipment, so make sure you use the exercises in the first six parts to strengthen your muscles before trying the trends exercises.

After you learn all of the weight-lifting exercises, you may wonder how you can combine them to create a routine you can follow during the week. In the last part of the book, I've included two-, three-, and four-day routines, as well as routines for muscle gain, weight loss, and 15-minute full-body work. Each gives you a sample routine you can follow, as well as information on how each routine is put together so you can adapt it to your own needs.

With the knowledge you gain from this book, you'll be able to advance to any fitness challenge or regimen that may interest you. This is an investment in you, and the outcome is a happy and healthy life!

The Setup

Each exercise is broken down with full-color photos that show you how to do the exercise, as well as callouts that provide helpful information about your form. The exercises may also contain a warning, tip, or variation sidebar. Warning sidebars cover the common form mistakes made when doing these exercises. Tip sidebars provide a modification to the exercise to make it easier, whether it's a change to the equipment or your body placement. Variation sidebars show you how to make the exercise more challenging.

I've also provided in the top-left corner of each exercise a front and back view of the body with the muscles worked highlighted. The following is a blown-up version of what you'll see, with includes callouts for the different muscles in the body.

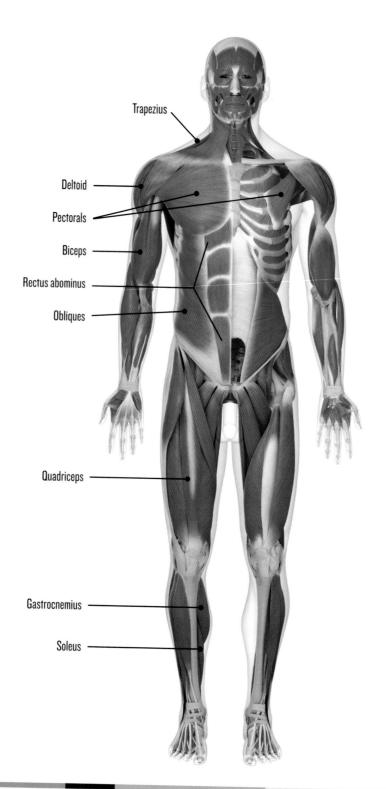

Trapezius

Deltoid

Pectorals

Biceps

Rectus abominus

Obliques

Quadriceps

Gastrocnemius

Soleus

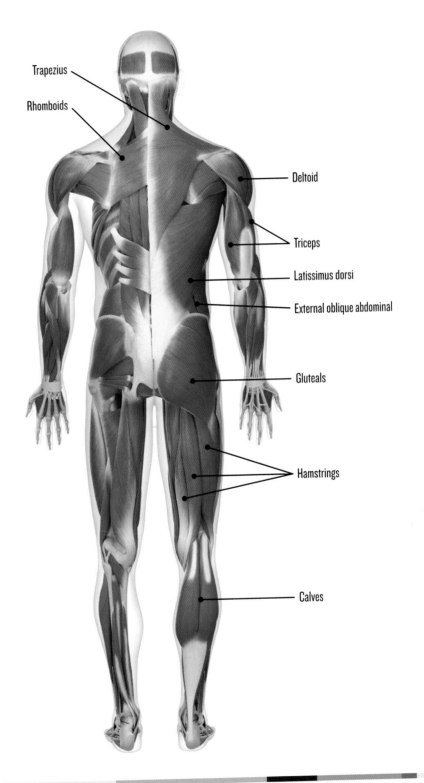

Trapezius

Rhomboids

Deltoid

Triceps

Latissimus dorsi

External oblique abdominal

Gluteals

Hamstrings

Calves

Acknowledgments

My mantra is "building hope, not just bodies." As a personal trainer, my goal is to bring a glimmer of hope into someone's life every day. Whether it be inside or outside of my training studio, without hope, we wouldn't work hard, try again, or open our hearts to give and receive love. My mother was very ill during the most demanding time of my writing, and I had to find the hope for her to be able to focus. Thank you, Lord, for letting her stay here with us! And thank you, Mom, for always believing in me to inspire and encourage others to be better every day.

I am so grateful for the inspiration and encouragement that I have received from all of the incredible people around me up to this point of my life. I have been extremely blessed to have parents that encouraged me, teachers and coaches that saw the potential in me and motivated me, and friends along the way that supported me. Now I have the best friend I could ever wish for, my husband Phil. Thank you all for being there for me and enriching my life!

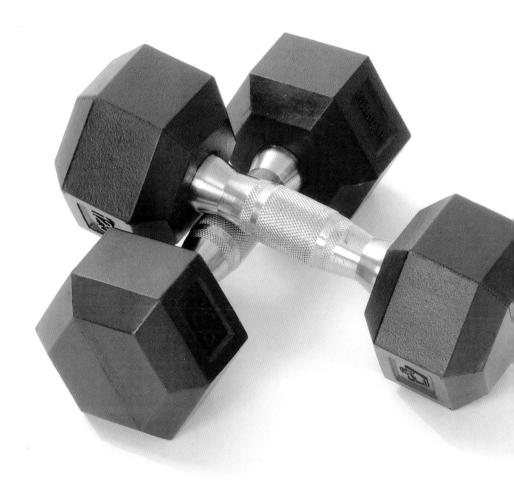

Weight Training Q&A

Q: What are the benefits of weight training?

A: Weight training is beneficial in many ways. By building new muscle and conditioning existing muscle, you'll keep your body in shape and improve your health. With more muscle, your body will also require more energy to run, which will increase your metabolism and make you a lean, mean, fat-burning machine. You'll even build stronger bones. When you lift weights or engage in other resistance-training activities, your bones are stimulated to become denser. And because your body will be in better shape and therefore performing at a higher level, you'll notice how much more alert you are during your daily routines.

Q: Should women stay away from lifting weights?

A: No! One misconception is that women won't look feminine if they lift weights. While it's possible for women to add a lot of visible muscle, it takes years and years of deliberate planning in terms of lifting, eating, and supplementation. But for women who just want to keep their muscles toned, lifting weights two to four times a week is a great way to look and feel good. Lifting weights can also boost metabolism or maintain a high metabolism in the body. Most women think their metabolism drops once they hit their 30s or 40s, when in reality, it doesn't just automatically drop. The slowing is most likely caused by women becoming less active as they age, meaning they're not using the muscle that fuels their metabolism. By lifting weights, women can stay active and keep their metabolism functioning at a high level.

Q: What are "free weights"?

A: The term *free weights* most commonly refers to dumbbells, barbells, and the plates that go on barbells. Using free weights recruits more stabilizing muscles than most exercise machines. For example, when you use a shoulder press machine, you sit on a stable seat with your back supported and press a bar attached to the machine. But when you perform a shoulder press with a set of dumbbells in each hand while sitting on a weight bench without any back support, you fire your core muscles and stabilize your arms individually. This book walks you through how to properly use all the different types of free weights.

Q: Is it better to do free weights or machines?

A: It is good to do both free weights and machines—both have their place in weight training. Your body requires more work and overall control to lift free weights because you aren't supported by the set structure of a machine. On the other hand, having the structure of a machine is a great way to learn proper form if you haven't had instruction on how to lift weights before. To say which one is better is tough. However, free weights are the most effective because you have to work harder and use more muscles to move them.

Q: Is it true that heavier weights and low reps build muscle while lighter weights and high reps tone muscle?

A: This is a big misconception in the weight-lifting world that keeps many people from pushing themselves out of fear of bulking up too much. The truth is that to build or tone muscle, you must break down the muscle. The science behind this phenomenon is that the muscle breaks, causing soreness; then, with proper recovery time, the muscle repairs and heals itself so it can grow. So if you want to tone up the muscle you already have or build muscle of any size, you must cause stress to the muscle to change your body. However, there's one big thing to keep in mind while lifting weights—*intensity!* You must challenge yourself. If you lift light weight for a high number of reps but don't "feel" anything the next day or the day after, you most likely didn't break down the muscle. On the other hand, you should only consider using the heaviest weight for low repetitions if you're going for a personal record. This is a common goal for power lifters and some body builders, but for a generally conditioned person who lifts weights for their health and fitness, this type of training is unnecessary and potentially harmful.

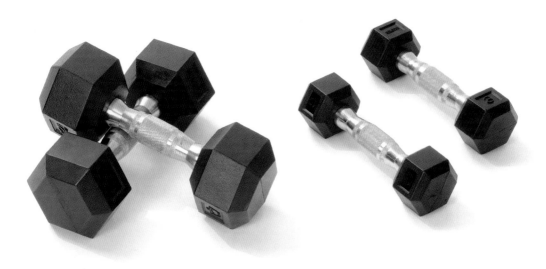

Q: How do I choose the proper weight for each exercise to start with?

A: Choosing the right weight to start with for each exercise can be tricky. For starters, it's always best to be smart and modest in your weight selection. Pick a weight you feel comfortable with, and complete a few full repetitions before you decide to either stay at that weight or trade the weight for another. To be sure you don't injure yourself in the process, it's better to have to go up to a heavier weight than down to a lighter weight. Also, if you find yourself cheating on proper form because the weight is too heavy, move down in weight so you can get the full range of motion and benefit out of a certain exercise. The more you lift weights, the quicker and more accurate your guess will be.

Q: How do I know when to move up in weights?

A: You may find yourself lifting the same amount of weight workout after workout simply out of habit. To know whether you need to move up in weights, pay attention to how you feel once you've completed a set. If you feel as if you could do 5 or more reps, it's time to move up. Also, remember that you need to use your workout time effectively. If you use the same weight on a certain exercise and just add reps as you go, it could get a little ridiculous in terms of time spent. Plus, it doesn't do you much good to use a weight that's light enough to make the first 10 reps super easy.

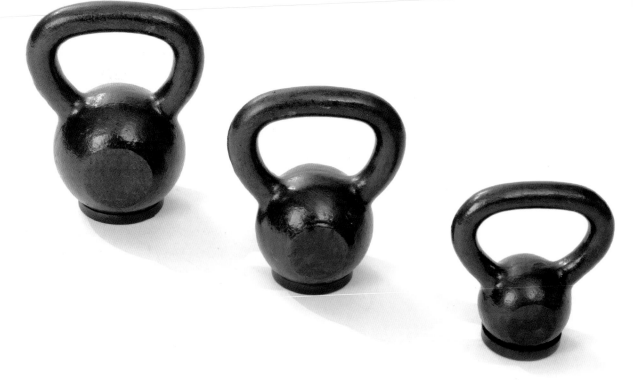

Q: What are kettlebells? Is kettlebell training a replacement for weight training?

A: Kettlebells are dense, cast-iron weights that resemble cannonballs with handles. Unlike a dumbbell, the bulk of the weight in a kettlebell is extended down past the hand. Kettlebells are very fun to train with, as long as you know what you're doing. Kettlebell training is very different than weight training in terms of technique and execution. While lifting weights requires control and precise placement, kettlebells bring a much more intense and explosive feel by using momentum to perform exercises.

Before you jump into using kettlebells, you should have a foundation of core strength and functional conditioning from weights, because you use multiple joints while doing full-body training during the movements. When you begin using kettlebells, you can take a break from your normal weight-lifting routine; however, kettlebells shouldn't replace traditional weight lifting in your regimen.

Q: What are suspension bands? Is suspension band training better for a beginner than weight training?

A: Suspension band training systems use your body weight and gravity to give you a full-body workout by simply using unstable straps that are mounted from the ceiling. In suspension band training, you not only use the major muscles to perform a certain movement, you recruit all of the stabilizers around them. While suspension bands can be used by people at every level of fitness, it's still very smart to have a good knowledge base of how your muscles work and a solid amount of conditioning before you attempt this challenging type of training. Because you're also engaging the stabilizers, it can be a great shock to the body if you're used to sitting or standing on a solid surface to perform your exercises.

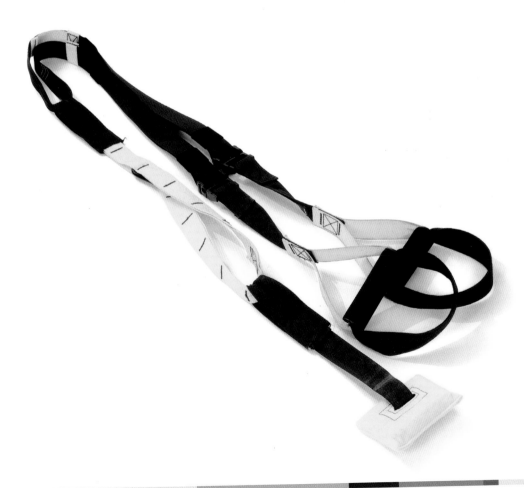

Q: Is it okay to lift weights every day?

A: It's completely fine to lift weights every day; however, doing so may be a bit difficult to plan. If you decide to lift every day, you must schedule your lifts in an order that allows your muscles to recover. Some muscle groups use the muscles from another group as secondary movers—for example, the chest press uses the pecs as the primary mover and triceps as the secondary mover to finish the movement. Therefore, it's smart to plan out your upper-body days away from each other to give your muscles plenty of time to recover. And because you'll only be able to focus on one muscle group a day, the routines may get boring or redundant.

Q: How long do my lifting routines need to be?

A: When lifting weights, you should always lift with purpose. This means having a plan to follow to keep you moving so you don't end up spending hours and hours in the gym at a time. A safe amount of time to allot for your weight lifting is anywhere from 25 to 55 minutes, depending on your level of conditioning and the length of the exercises. Much more than an hour of weights is unnecessary and could lead to too much soreness and possibly injury.

Q: How many days a week should I work out?

A: You don't need to work out a certain number of days a week—after all, one day in the gym is better than none at all. However, no matter how many days you can devote to lifting weights, it helps to have a plan. A solid plan will cover every muscle in the body, with each workout complementing the next, and will allow your muscles proper rest between workouts.

Q: If I only have two days a week that I can commit to the gym, is that enough?

A: Most definitely. When it comes to working out, don't limit yourself to an all-or-nothing mentality. If you do, you won't get very far with your fitness goals. Two days a week gives you plenty of time to have a balanced and adequate amount of weight lifting. On a two-day schedule, be sure to keep your intensity up and move quickly through the routines. While you may think you should double or triple the time you spend working out because you aren't in the gym every day, that's unnecessary. Just make sure you choose exercises that will maximize your time spent.

Q: When is the best time of the day to work out?

A: The best time of the day to work out is when you have time! If you make it a priority to set time aside in your busy day to work out, that's great; however, don't worry too much about finding the right time to do it. If you tend to be wired after a workout, it's a good idea to start early in the day rather than at night—otherwise, you might have trouble sleeping. Working out earlier also turns on your metabolism earlier in the day. If you have a house full of kids and a spouse to take care of, a workout during your lunch break may be the answer. If you normally work out in the morning but feel run down, sleep in and work out that evening. Your body will let you know when it needs rest; it will beg for it, if you don't pick up on the hints! If you simply don't have time to get to the gym or work out at home one day, don't stress out. There's always a fresh new opportunity the next day to build a stronger body!

Q: What is the difference between reps and sets?

A: Reps and sets help you chart how long your workout is and the number of times you do the exercises. "Reps" is short for *repetitions;* it's the number of times you do a specific exercise or movement at one time. "Sets" refers to the total number of reps as a whole. So, for example, "3 sets of 15" means you would do 15 reps for 3 rounds. You may also see sets and reps written with a times sign between them—for example, 3×15.

Q: What is a superset?

A: A superset is when you perform different exercises back to back without a rest in between. You can create a superset that challenges the same muscle group in a different way. For example, you can do a chest press and a chest fly in the same set; the chest fly provides a bigger stretch to the pecs than you'd get just doing the chest press. You can also do a superset that works one muscle group before challenging another muscle group, giving that first group a rest. For example, you may try performing a chest press with a chest fly, followed by a shoulder press.

Q: How many sets and reps should I do during each exercise?

A: A good range to shoot for in terms of reps is 10 to 12. You'll know within the first 3 to 5 reps of a specific movement whether you have the right weight for your fitness level. If you feel you could do 20 more reps with the weight, it's most likely time to move up to a heavier weight; if you're already feeling like you can't continue on, you need a lighter weight. Sometimes, you should change up your rep range, just like you would change up your routines; doing this keeps your muscles guessing.

The proper amount of sets to perform can vary. When doing a new routine, you may want to start with 1 to 2 sets, then add a third set after a couple weeks, depending on how your body feels. In some cases, you may even want to do more than 3 sets to train for muscle endurance by pushing past the normal amount of reps that you're used to.

However, keep in mind that it is completely fine to scale your sets or reps back a notch if you feel that you have set the number too high. For example, if you have a goal to perform a set of push-ups for 10 reps but feel your form breaking by the sixth push-up, you should stop to prevent injury. It all comes down to having a plan and knowing your body.

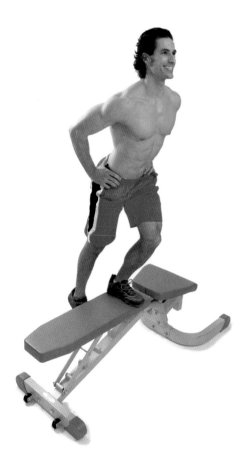

Q: What is the difference between simple and compound exercises?

A: The joints and muscles involved in a specific exercise determine the difference between a simple and a compound exercise. For example, the bicep curl is a simple (or isolation) exercise because you're hinging at one joint, the elbow, to perform the exercise. Simple exercises are nice for rehabbing an injury or simply getting a nice pump to one smaller muscle group during a workout. An example of a compound movement would be a squat, because your hip and knee joints are flexing and extending to work your quads, hamstrings, and glutes. Compound movements are used in many sports and weight-lifting workouts because they condition the full body.

Q: How many exercises per muscle group should I do in a workout?

A: Because each exercise has its own set of benefits (such as a certain stretch or hold), you'll find it very helpful to incorporate many different exercises per muscle group as you progress your workout routines. When you are starting out with weight training, pick one to two exercises per muscle group. Later, you can add more exercises in order to continue breaking down and fatiguing the muscles. However, try not to add too soon. If you do, go ahead and drop back down to the previous number of exercises you were doing for the muscle group.

Q: Is it possible to do a full-body workout every time I work out?

A: It is possible to do a full-body workout every time you train; however, you would also have to have many days of rest and recovery in between workouts. If you want, you can choose different exercises to do every four or five days. These workouts could be a "full-body" workout without doing the same exact routine. For example, you could do a squat, chest press, and tricep extension for day 1, and a deadlift, pull-up, and bicep curl for day 2. The days are considered full-body because you're working your lower and upper body together in one workout and still doing different exercises. Also, in the example, you have all "pushing" movements on day 1 and all "pulling" movements on day 2; this allows the muscles to complement each other in the routines. And instead of having to spend hours in the gym to try to cover all these exercises in one routine, having a split like this will help keep your workout time bearable.

Q: What is the best exercise to burn fat?

A: Muscles are the number-one driver of metabolism. The more muscle you have, the more fat you'll burn, giving you a leaner physique. Therefore, you should choose exercises that work your major muscles first, such as squats, deadlifts, pull-ups, and push-ups. These exercises are very powerful in working the whole body so you become leaner and stronger.

Q: How long should I rest between sets and exercises?

A: A nice way to manage your rests is to watch the clock and give yourself 30 to 60 seconds to rest in between sets. As you progress your workouts and step up the intensity, you can take shorter rests. With shorter rest periods, you're asking the body to recover quicker. That's not an easy task, or something you can just decide to do! Therefore, you'll need to be smart about timing your rest out—make sure you allow yourself enough time for your heart rate to come down and your muscles to relax.

Q: How many days should I rest between workouts?

A: There's no set amount of time you should rest between workouts—just remember that the muscle needs to heal and recover completely before being used (broken down) again. Start with a once-a-week lifting schedule for each muscle group to be certain you give them enough recovery time. As you become more aware of your muscles and how they respond to lifting weights, you can shorten the rest in between workouts.

If you don't allow your muscles enough time to recover, your body will start to shut down the drive and power you initially felt when you started lifting weights. You may think that your enthusiasm or eagerness has dropped, when in reality your body is *making* you stop. This is most commonly called *overtraining*. Some signs that you're approaching overtraining are: loss of appetite, lack of energy, restless sleep or trouble falling asleep, weakness or fainting spells during nonexercise activities, carelessness (lack of attention or recklessness), and a sense of memory loss. But don't let these symptoms scare you. As long as you put careful thought into planning your workouts and allow your body to rest in between, you'll be just fine.

Q: What does it mean to hit a plateau? How do I know if I have hit a plateau?

A: A plateau is hit when your muscles are no longer challenged by a certain exercise or type of training. When your body gets used to doing a specific activity like running, swimming, or even weight lifting, it isn't as demanding and in return may not be as beneficial to finding new fitness results. To get off the plateau, employ muscle confusion.

Q: What is muscle confusion?

A: Muscle confusion is when you vary your workout routines to avoid hitting a plateau, which comes from your body getting too used to a set routine. A few ways to employ muscle confusion are changing up the type of training style, intensity, length of the workout, or frequency.

Q: What are the core muscles?

A: Your core muscles surround your spine, ribs, and pelvis. People tend to assume core muscles refer to the abs, when in reality there are a lot more muscles that make up the core. Core muscles include your abdominals, obliques, spine erectors, and even lats (because of their ability to stabilize your torso while walking and sitting upright), just to name a few. Weight training will condition these muscles because they're always turned on to assist in exercises, especially if you're using free weights. Having strong core muscles will not only help you in weight lifting, it will also improve posture.

Q: Should I do cardio before or after lifting weights?

A: To avoid injury, it's a good idea to warm up your body before you begin lifting weights. This may include 5 to 10 minutes of light cardio to get your body temperature up and your muscles warm. If you do much more than that, the energy systems in the body will be depleted and you won't have the stamina and strength you need for lifting weights.

A nice form of cardio is walking on a treadmill with a slight incline. You can do 5 to 10 minutes of walking at a speed level of 3 to 4 and an incline level of 3.5 to 4. Ellipticals, cross trainers, stairmills, and bikes are also great for warming up before a weight-training workout—just make sure to keep the resistance low on these machines.

When doing light cardio, your heart rate should stay around 90 to 100 beats per minute. Most machines have a heart rate monitor on them, but if you need another way to know whether you're at the right level, see if you're able to hold a conversation. If you find yourself huffing and puffing for air, you're most likely pushing a little too hard for a warm-up.

Q: Should I stretch before or after a workout?

A: While it's smart to warm up before a workout, as far as stretching goes, it can be harmful to fully stretch out a muscle before asking it to push around weight. The act of lifting weights is about both stretching and contracting the muscle. If the muscle is already stretched out, it may not have the same amount of strength to perform an exercise that it would have without any warm-up stretching. A better way to get ready for a workout routine that won't fully stretch out the muscle is to perform a few warm-up reps or a full warm-up set with a very light weight or even your bodyweight. That way, you can prepare your muscles for what's coming before you pick up the actual weight you plan to use during the workout.

Q: What is the best thing to eat before and after I lift weights?

A: Think of everything you eat as fuel that can either help or hinder your fitness goals. Before and after you lift weights, your body needs energy. Choose unprocessed and natural sources of carbohydrates, such as oatmeal, brown rice, grains like quinoa or amaranth, and all vegetables and fruits. Also, be sure to get protein into your diet by eating chicken, eggs, and fish and supplementing with whey powder. The carbs will refuel the energy stores depleted during your workout. The protein—and the amino acids supplied by them—will help your muscles start the recovery process and give you energy.

Keep in mind that fat sources, although vital to your health, aren't the best to eat before or after a workout because they are slower digesting. Also, simple sugars from junk food or sodas are more of a hindrance than a help to a good workout because they are filled with empty calories. Stick with protein and carbs because you need the energy shuttled into your system quickly to support the workout.

Q: Should I avoid carbs if I'm trying to lose weight?

A: No, definitely not. If you don't have the proper energy to put into a workout, it's impossible to have the strength to work out at all, let alone lose weight. Carbs from natural sources—such as quinoa, brown rice, sprouted-grain breads, oatmeal, fruits, and vegetables—provide fuel for your brain and body so you can power through your workout. However, try to avoid processed carbs, such as pasta and bread—they can raise your blood sugar.

Q: Is it best to work out alone or with a partner?

A: When it comes to working out with a partner or rolling solo, it depends on what works best for you personally. In some settings, having a workout partner can bring a healthy amount of friendly competition and accountability, as you and your partner push each other to achieve your goals. For this arrangement to work, you should pick someone who is on the same fitness level as you, so one of you isn't struggling to keep up or being held back. Also, find someone who's focused on the task at hand.

If you have a regular workout partner, always be courteous when it comes to their time and your own. If one party isn't feeling like training, don't let it affect the other's motivation. Find the drive and motivation deep down so you don't solely rely on the other person to get to the gym. If you're in a time crunch or simply have goals that are different from potential workout partners, it may be best to work out alone.

Q: What is meant by "good form," and how to I achieve it?

A: Having good form is like having insurance on a prized possession. You want to be certain you get the benefit of each and every workout by learning the proper techniques to keep your form right. The goal of the step-by-step breakdown of the exercises in this book is to teach you how to have good form. When learning the exercises, take a close look at the models' body placement for each step. Also, check out the warnings about avoiding improper form, whether it's not letting your knees go past your toes or not letting your shoulders round down. You will most likely get sick of hearing me say these two things, but heeding the warnings will save you from potential injury and long-term pain!

Q: Would I benefit from a personal trainer?

A: No matter your fitness level, you can benefit from hiring a personal trainer. Think about it: The super-conditioned professional athletes? The Hollywood celebs with enviable bodies? Many, if not all of those people, have worked with a personal trainer. Even if it's only for a session or two, having the guidance of a personal trainer will make you feel confident about your exercises and technique. Also, finding a knowledgeable trainer who fits your personality can be very helpful along your fitness journey.

Q: What should I look for in a personal trainer?

A: Similar to looking for a barber, finding a trainer can be like flipping a coin—some folks get lucky and land on a perfect match for their personality and workout preferences, while others may have to meet with a few before they right one. Before you sign up to meet with anyone, though, it pays to do a little research. If your gym has a list of their personal trainers, look it over for names, contact information, and bios and credentials (if those are available). Another option is to find trainers who have something good to say about themselves! When you find a trainer that you are interested in working with, first check that person's schedule to make sure you have the same availability. If that works out, you can then schedule a consultation with the trainer. This is a very important step, because the consultation will act as a trial run to see how you and the trainer mesh.

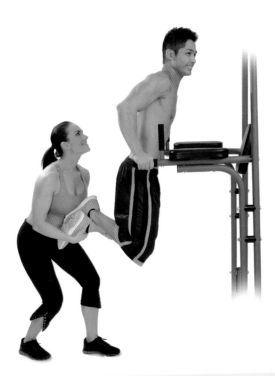

Q: What should I look for when choosing a gym to belong to?

A: You can find gyms that provide many different options, such as fitness classes, childcare, a pool, a sauna, a hot tub, a basketball court, or even special hours. When choosing a gym, decide what options are important to you and see whether they're part of the membership fee or cost extra. Do you want a full-service gym with all the amenities included? Or do you prefer something simpler, where you can just go and lift weights? Choose the gym that best fits your personal workout needs. If you end up deciding you don't like the gym you've chosen, you can always look for another one.

Q: What does "gym etiquette" mean?

A: You demonstrate proper gym etiquette by showing respect to the equipment and the other gym members around you. When you're finished with your weights, it's proper etiquette to always re-rack them. By cleaning up and returning the weights to their proper place, you not only make it easier for the next person to find the equipment, you also give that person the green light to begin using it. If you've sweat on the equipment or machine, clean it off. Most gyms provide sanitation for wiping down your machine or equipment once you're done using it, but make sure you also have a towel on hand.

Q: What type of clothes and shoes should I wear at the gym?

A: When picking out what you'll wear at the gym, don't think about what's most fashionable or how other people are dressed; instead, think about what will be most comfortable for you as you work out. Some people like airy, loose-fitting clothes, while others may prefer tight-fitting workout gear that can wick away sweat and won't get in the way—it's 100 percent personal preference. The same goes with shoes. You can choose from hundreds of different types of tennis shoes, so look for ones that are comfortable and support your feet. Just think: no one has been kicked out of the gym for wearing the wrong clothes (well, maybe for not wearing *enough* clothes!).

Q: Is it okay to wear headphones at the gym?

A: Wearing headphones while working out is very common and is considered proper etiquette. Some folks may wear headphones to keep their focus and motivation up. Others may do it to block out distractions, such as overhead music or others around them. Just be sure you're courteous and pay attention to others around you, because wearing headphones can seem to put you in your own little world. Don't turn your music up so loud that you're unapproachable in the gym; keep it low enough that someone can speak to you in regard to sharing a piece of equipment or when you might be done using it.

Q: When do I need a spotter at the gym?

A: You only need a spotter when you aren't certain you'll be able to complete a set with the weight you're lifting. Consider having someone spot you when you're doing big power movements—like squats or chest and shoulder presses—with a heavy weight over your head. Another time you might need a spotter is when you're doing bodyweight pull-ups and dips; this person can act as "buddy assistance" for the little bit of help you may need to complete the movement. If you can't find anyone to spot you, skip the exercise. If you take the risk of not having a spotter when you need one, you could put yourself in a dangerous position! There's plenty of time to get those exercises in, so be patient and smart.

Q: Is it okay to ask a stranger at the gym to spot me?

A: If you're working out alone and find yourself needing a spotter, it's perfectly fine to ask a stranger nearby to spot you. Most weight lifters will quickly jump at the opportunity to help you out, as they understand the importance of proper form while lifting. Try to ask at a time when the person seems to be in between sets themselves, so you aren't interrupting his or her workout. Making friends and getting to know certain familiar faces builds a sense of respect and camaraderie at the gym, so that when they need a spotter, they know they can come to you!

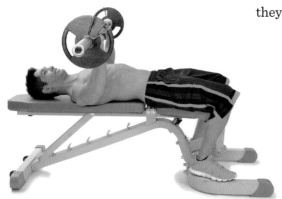

Q: How do I build a home gym?

A: Building a home gym can be a very convenient way to work out, and you don't need much to get started. Depending on the amount of space you have to work with, start with a few staple and versatile pieces of equipment, such as a weight bench, a set of 10-pound dumbbells, and a set of 20-pound dumbbells. With a lighter and heavier set of dumbbells, you'll have your bases covered for most exercises. A few other items that give you a big bang for your buck are a stability ball, resistance bands, and a suspension band trainer. These pieces of equipment take up very little space and offer tons of different ways to work out.

Q: How soon will I see results?

A: Everyone's body responds to weight lifting at different rates. A few things will determine how soon you might see a change in your body: age, body composition (how much body fat you have), diet, and frequency of workouts. The hard part of any workout regimen is sticking with it. It's important to know that while you may not visually see the changes right away, your body is still benefiting from lifting weights. Patience is key. If you stay dedicated and give it time, you'll wake up one morning and realize you've built an incredible body. As you work out, think of the difference you'll see in your body after a week, a month, and even a year of sticking to your plan, as well as how happy you'll be with the results. It will blow your mind!

You can also keep track of your progress in a training log. By writing down your routines and results as you go, you'll have a nice reference in which you can look up all your numbers and goals hit. You can even set future goals along the way!

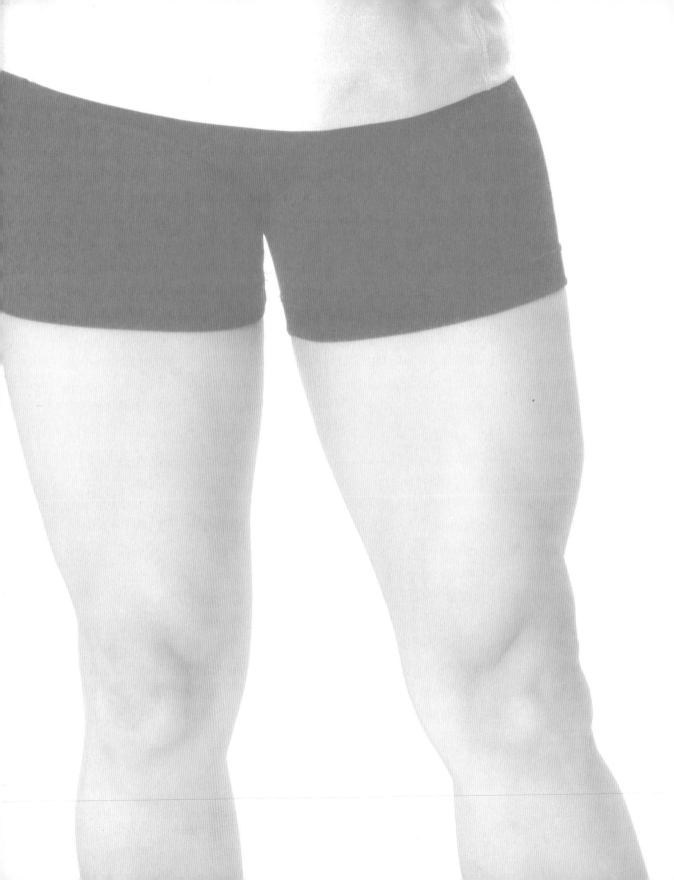

LEGS
(Glutes, Quads, Hamstrings, and Calves)

Weight training the muscles in your legs is like building a solid foundation for your home. Your legs are made up of the largest muscles in your body and can handle a lot, considering you use them every day; therefore, they require some good, hard time to become strong and powerful.

Your gluteals or **glutes** are the strongest muscles per surface area in your entire body; their primary function is to extend your hips and move your legs away from your body. Your glutes are very important to train because they're actively recruited in even the smallest movements, such as lowering yourself down to sit on a chair. Your quadriceps or **quads** are in the front of your thigh and are activated every time you extend your legs. On the opposite side of the leg are your **hamstrings,** which are the muscles responsible for pulling or flexing, making them vital to your everyday movement. Your **calves** are made up of the soleus and gastrocnemius muscles. They are used when you walk to stabilize each step.

Conditioning the muscles in your legs will not only give you a head-turning physique, it will also boost your metabolism and energy levels. And because your legs are your foundation, you'll be less likely to have back pain or injury when your lower body is strong.

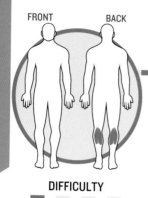

FRONT BACK

DIFFICULTY

Standing Calf Raise

The standing calf raise is a very simple exercise that's nice to include in your lower-body routine—think of it as a stretch as well as a strengthener for your gastrocnemius and soleus muscles (calves). Because you use your calves so much throughout the day, they will thank you for showing them some attention.

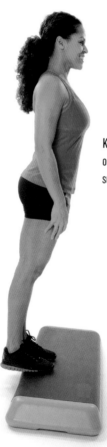

Keep your balance by holding on to a bar or the wall for support.

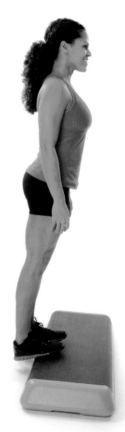

1 Stand on the edge of a step with only the balls of your feet and toes.

2 Inhale as you lower your heels below your toes to stretch your calves.

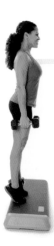

Variation
To progress this exercise, hold a weight down by your side. Try using a dumbbell or plate in one hand while the other keeps balance on a bar or wall, or hold weights in both hands.

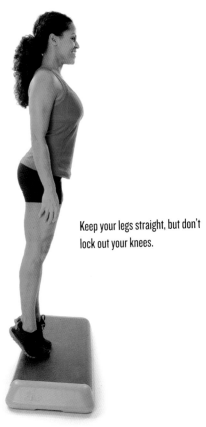

Keep your legs straight, but don't lock out your knees.

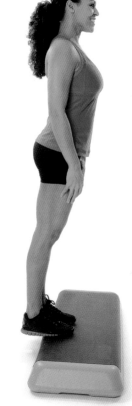

 3 Exhale as you raise your heels up past your toes. Squeeze your calves tight at the top of your extension.

4 Inhale as you descend back to starting position.

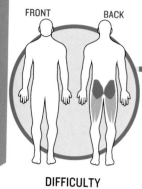

FRONT BACK

Bridge

The hip extension in the bridge is involved in nearly every lower-body movement, making it a simple yet very important exercise. It targets your gluteals (butt) and hamstrings (back of your legs).

DIFFICULTY

1 Lie on your back and allow your knees to bend. Keep your feet flat on the floor.

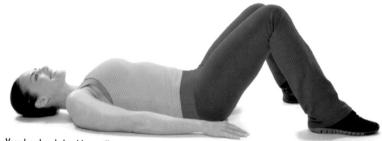

Your head and shoulders will rest on the floor for the entire exercise.

Keep your abs engaged.

2 Exhale as you press through your heels up into the bridge.

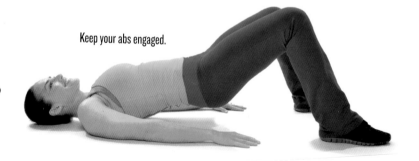

Adjust the height of the bridge by putting your feet up on a step or even a bench.

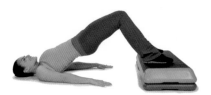

Variation
Give yourself an added challenge by using a stability ball at your feet. You can put your arms and hands out to your sides on the floor for balance.

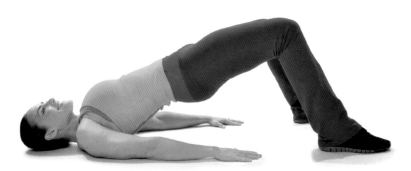

3 Once you are fully in the bridge position, pause and hold it for a moment.

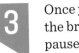

You can use support from your hands as they rest on the floor down at your sides.

4 Inhale as you return back to starting position.

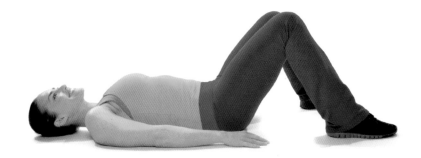

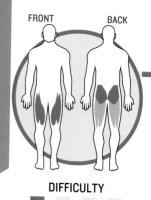

FRONT   BACK

DIFFICULTY

Bodyweight Squat

The squat is an essential movement in weight lifting. It mimics a simple action you complete multiple times a day—sitting down and standing up from a chair—yet it targets many muscles in your lower body, including your gluteals (butt), quadriceps (thighs), and hamstrings (back of your legs).

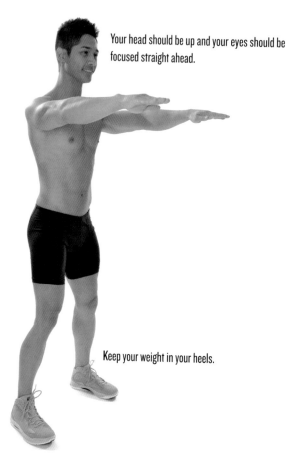

Your head should be up and your eyes should be focused straight ahead.

Keep your weight in your heels.

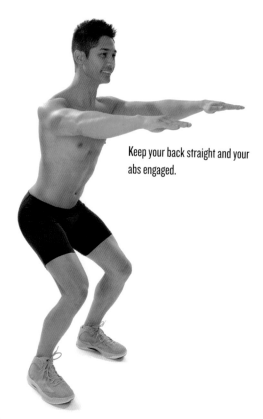

Keep your back straight and your abs engaged.

1 Stand with your feet shoulder width apart. If you like, you may have your arms out for balance.

2 Rock your hips back to create a natural arch in your back. Keeping your weight in your heels, inhale as you squat down.

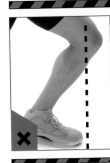

Be Careful!
Don't allow your knees to go past your toes. Doing so could cause injury due to too much pressure on your joints.

Practice the squat position by lowering yourself down to sit on a chair or bench. This allows you to feel the proper form—with your weight shifted onto your heels—as your muscles control you down, then back up.

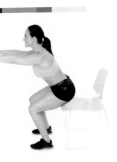

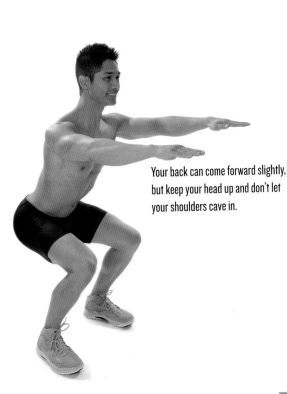

Your back can come forward slightly, but keep your head up and don't let your shoulders cave in.

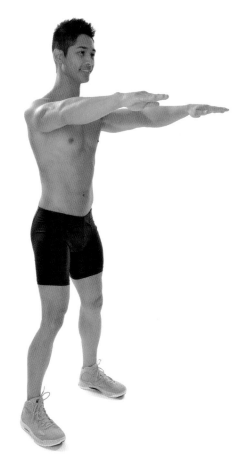

3 At the bottom of the squat, your legs should be at a 90-degree angle.

4 Exhale as you rise back to starting position.

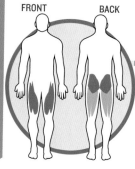

FRONT   BACK

DIFFICULTY

Bodyweight Lunge

The lunge challenges your balance and strengthens your posture. Although it may seem like a simple exercise, it's often done with poor form. With proper technique, this exercise works your quadriceps (thighs), gluteals (butt), and hamstrings (back of your legs).

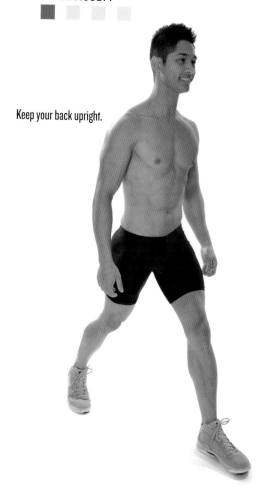

Keep your back upright.

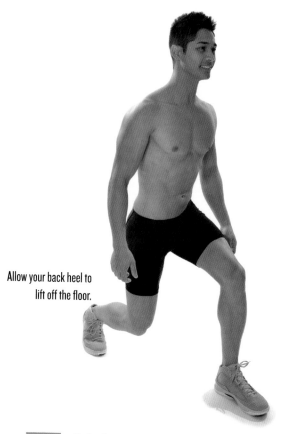

Allow your back heel to lift off the floor.

1 Stand with one foot in front of the other, with your weight equally balanced between the two.

2 Inhale as you lower into the lunge.

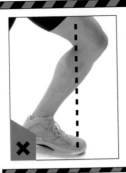

Be Careful!
Always watch out for your knee joints, as the pressure on the joints is too great if they're bent past the 90-degree angle. Allowing your knees to go past your toes may cause long-term pain and serious injury.

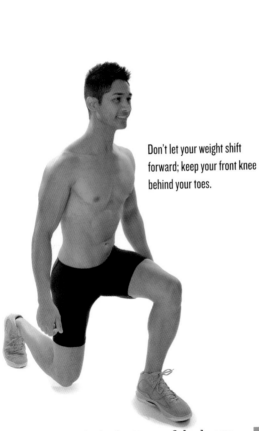

Don't let your weight shift forward; keep your front knee behind your toes.

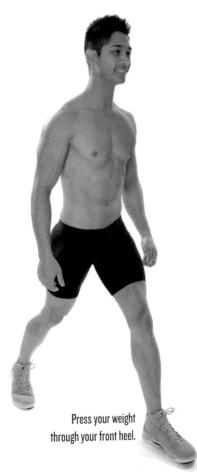

Press your weight through your front heel.

3 Once you reach the bottom of the lunge, your legs should be at 90-degree angles.

4 Exhale as you rise back to starting position.

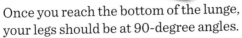

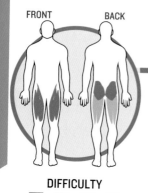

FRONT   BACK

Sumo Squat

The wide stance of the sumo squat gives your inner thighs a nice stretch. It targets the major muscles of your lower body, including your gluteals (butt), hamstrings (back of your legs), and quadriceps (thighs).

DIFFICULTY

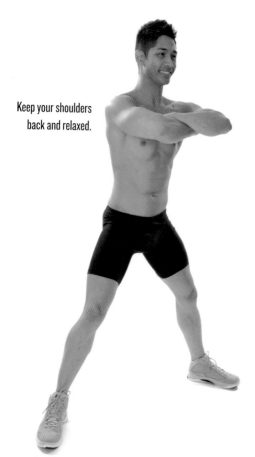

Keep your shoulders back and relaxed.

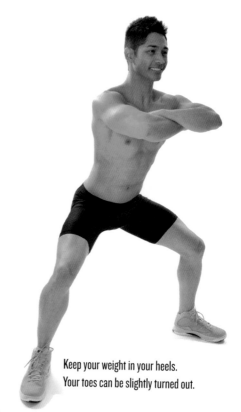

Keep your weight in your heels.
Your toes can be slightly turned out.

1 Stand with your feet outside of your shoulders for a strong, wide stance.

2 Rock your hips back for a natural tilt in your pelvis. Inhale as you squat down.

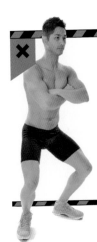

Be Careful!
Like the bodyweight squat, be careful to not let your knees go out past your toes. Always be aware of the angles in your joints to protect them from injury.

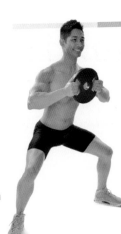

Variation
To provide extra work for your core and lower body, hold a weight at your chest or near the center of your body. You can use a medicine ball, a barbell plate, or even a dumbbell.

Keep your eyes up to protect your lower back from arching.

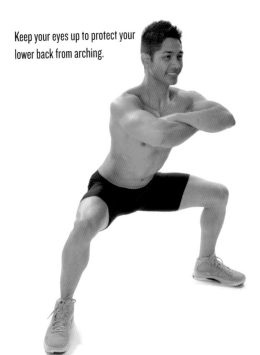

3 At the bottom of the squat, your legs should be at a 90-degree angle.

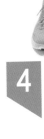

4 Exhale as you ascend back to starting position.

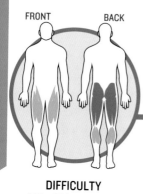

FRONT   BACK

Stability Ball Hamstring Curl

Similar to the bridge, this exercise works your glutes and hamstrings. By adding a stability ball, you challenge your balance.

DIFFICULTY

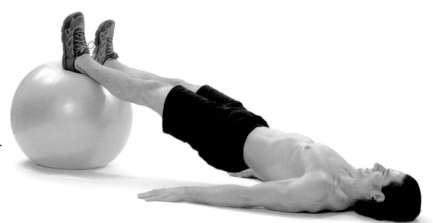

1 With both feet on the stability ball, bridge your body off the floor and inhale as you find balance.

Your upper body should rest on the floor for the entire exercise.

Keep your feet firmly planted on the ball.

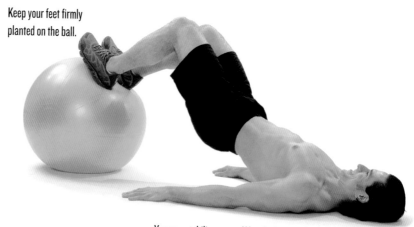

2 Keep your body lifted and exhale as you roll your ankles in toward your butt.

You can stabilize yourself by placing your hands at your sides on the floor.

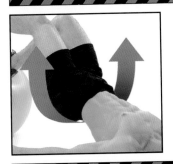

Be Careful!
During this exercise, make sure your hips stay up. Otherwise, your calves will do the work that your hamstrings and glutes should be doing.

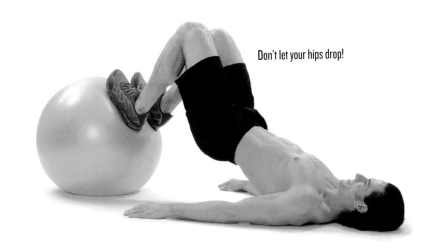

Don't let your hips drop!

3 Roll in until your knees are at a 90-degree angle.

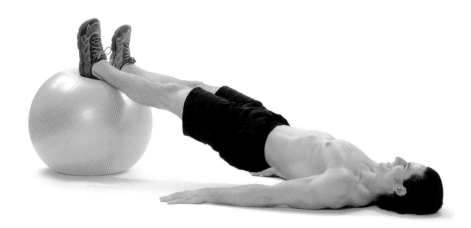

4 Inhale as you roll the ball back out to straight legs and return to starting position.

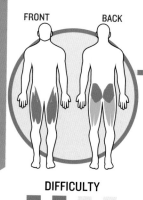

FRONT   BACK

DIFFICULTY

Step-Up

The step-up is one of the most effective yet underrated exercises for your lower body. It seems as simple as walking up a flight of stairs, but when you step up onto a much higher step with proper form in mind, you get a more beneficial exercise that sculpts your legs. This exercise targets your quads and glutes.

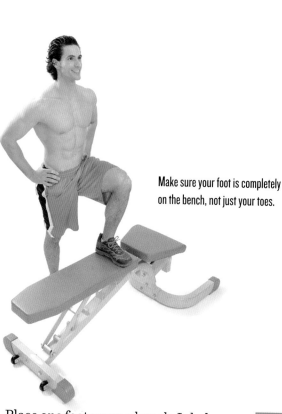

Make sure your foot is completely on the bench, not just your toes.

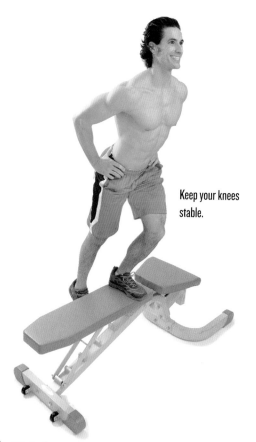

Keep your knees stable.

1 Place one foot up on a bench. Inhale as you prepare to step up.

2 Exhale as you step up to the top of the bench.

Be Careful!

It is very important to keep proper form while doing this exercise. Don't think the higher the step, the harder the exercise. If the step is too high, you may not use the correct muscles and could even hurt yourself.

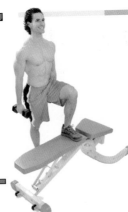

Variation

For an extra challenge to your core and your lower body, hold dumbbells down at your sides while performing this exercise. Keep your form in mind and choose a weight that will not pull your shoulders forward.

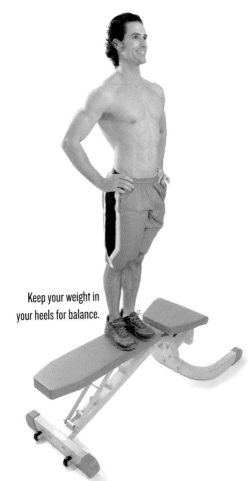

Keep your weight in your heels for balance.

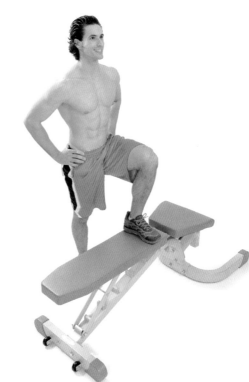

3 Squeeze your glutes at the top of the movement. Be sure to finish straightening the leg that started on the bench before your other foot reaches the bench.

4 Inhale as you descend back to starting position.

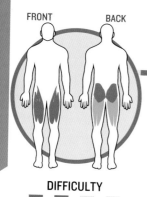

FRONT   BACK

Lateral Lunge

This version of the lunge incorporates a great deal of balance and gives your inner thighs a nice stretch. It targets the major muscles of your lower body, including your glutes, hamstrings, and quads.

DIFFICULTY

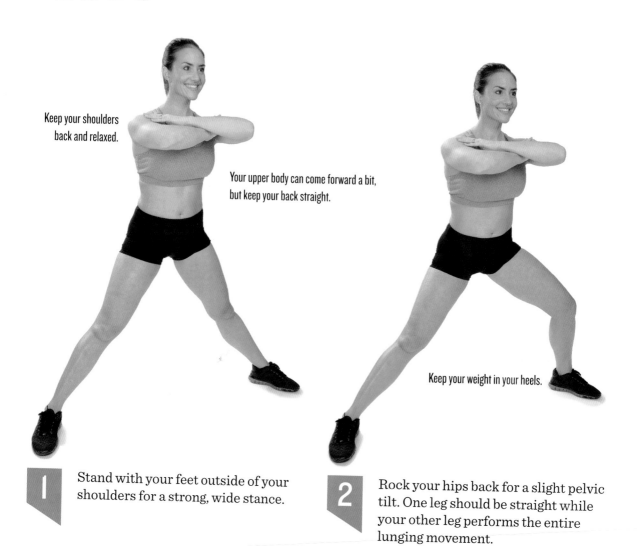

Keep your shoulders back and relaxed.

Your upper body can come forward a bit, but keep your back straight.

Keep your weight in your heels.

1 Stand with your feet outside of your shoulders for a strong, wide stance.

2 Rock your hips back for a slight pelvic tilt. One leg should be straight while your other leg performs the entire lunging movement.

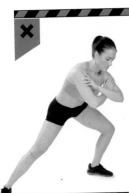

Be Careful!

Watch your form during the lunge. To avoid injury, keep your toes and knees facing forward, and don't let your knee extend past your toes.

Variation

Add weight to your lateral lunge by holding a plate or medicine ball at chest level. This will incorporate more work for your core muscles while challenging your lower body to support more weight during the lunge.

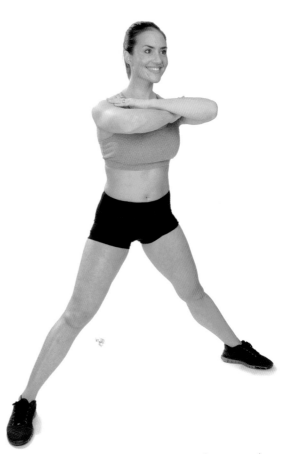

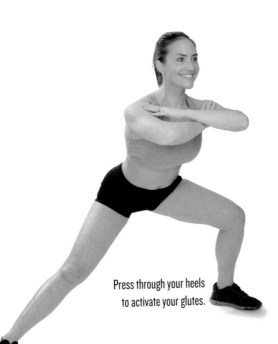

Press through your heels to activate your glutes.

3 Inhale as your lunging leg lowers down to one side. You should feel the inner-thigh stretch of the straight leg.

4 Exhale as you ascend back to starting position.

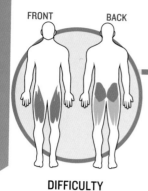

FRONT   BACK

Dumbbell Squat

To progress from the bodyweight squat, you can hold dumbbells for added weight. This exercise works the major muscles in your legs, including your quads, glutes, and hamstrings. You also build your core and upper-body stability with the dumbbells.

DIFFICULTY

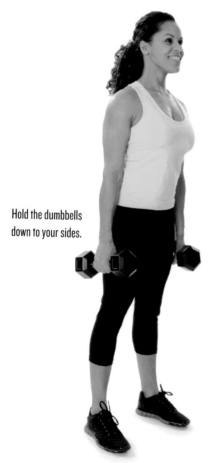

Hold the dumbbells down to your sides.

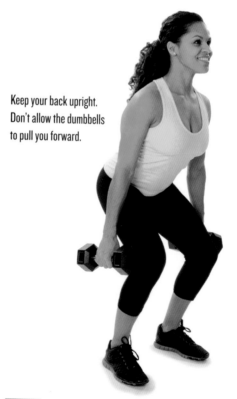

Keep your back upright. Don't allow the dumbbells to pull you forward.

1 Stand with your feet shoulder width apart. Keep your bodyweight in your heels.

2 Rock your hips back to create a natural arch in your back. Inhale and squat down.

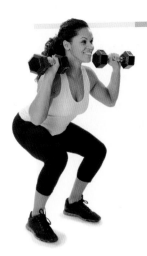

Variation

To incorporate your core even more in this exercise, bring the dumbbells to your shoulders. Don't allow the dumbbells to rest on your shoulders or pull you forward. This move will prepare you for upper body-loaded squats (such as front squats) or back-loaded squats with a barbell.

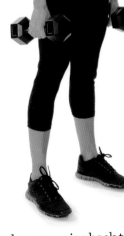

Maintain your posture as you come back up.

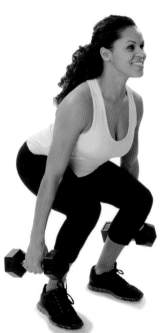

Keep your arms down to your sides, with a comfortable grip on the dumbbells.

3 At the bottom of the squat, your legs should be at a 90-degree angle.

4 Exhale as you rise back to starting position.

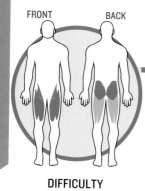

FRONT BACK

LEGS

DIFFICULTY

Dumbbell Lunge

To progress from the bodyweight lunge, you can hold dumbbells for added weight. Choose a weight that allows you to keep proper form yet challenges you. This movement works the major muscles in your legs, including your quads, glutes, and hamstrings. The addition of dumbbells also helps you build your core and upper-body stability.

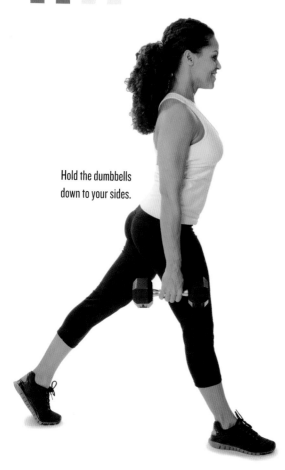

Hold the dumbbells down to your sides.

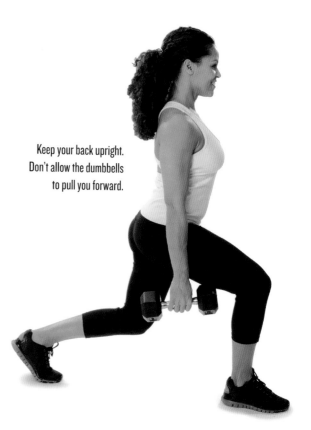

Keep your back upright. Don't allow the dumbbells to pull you forward.

1 Stand with one foot in front of the other, with your weight equally balanced between the two. Allow your back heel to lift.

2 Inhale and lower into the lunge.

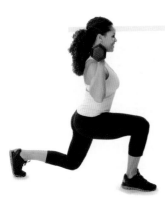

Variation

To incorporate your core even more in this exercise, bring the dumbbells to your shoulders. Just make sure the dumbbells don't rest on your shoulders or pull you forward.

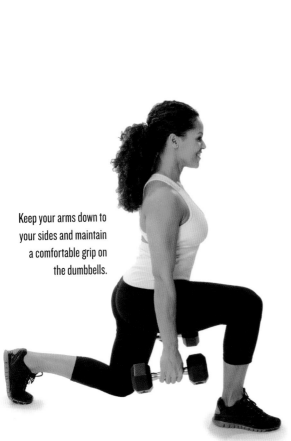

Keep your arms down to your sides and maintain a comfortable grip on the dumbbells.

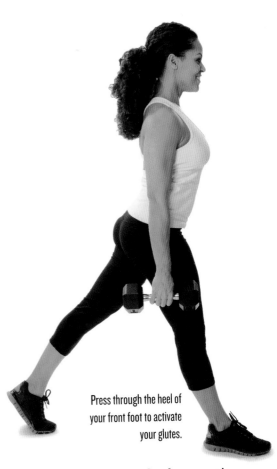

Press through the heel of your front foot to activate your glutes.

3 Pause before your knee reaches the floor. Your legs should be at 90-degree angles.

4 Exhale as you rise back to starting position.

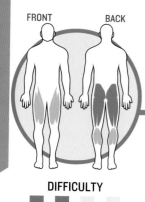

FRONT   BACK

DIFFICULTY

Stability Ball Single-Leg Hamstring Curl

Challenge your balance even more by doing the hamstring curl one leg at a time. The leg not performing the exercise will float up and out of the way, allowing your supporting leg to do all the work! This exercise targets your glutes and hamstrings.

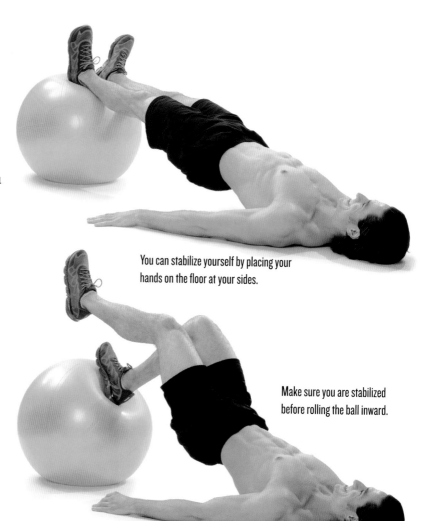

1 With your feet on the stability ball, bridge your body off of the floor and inhale as you find balance.

You can stabilize yourself by placing your hands on the floor at your sides.

2 Keep your body lifted and exhale as you lift one foot off the stability ball. With the foot still on the stability ball, roll your ankle in toward your butt.

Make sure you are stabilized before rolling the ball inward.

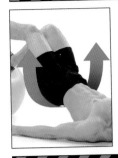

Be Careful!
Don't allow your hips to drop during this move. If you feel less work from your hamstrings and glutes, most likely your calves have taken over because your hips have lowered down. Keep those hips up, even when there's only one leg doing all the work!

Keep the foot doing the movement firmly planted on the ball.

3 Roll until your leg doing the curl on the ball forms a 90-degree angle in the knee, while your other leg lifts straight into the air.

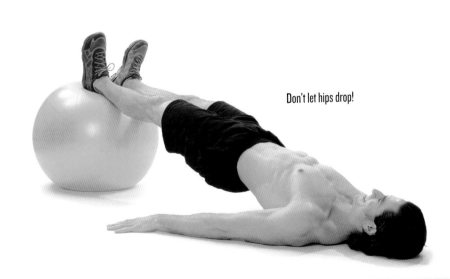

Don't let hips drop!

4 Inhale as you roll the ball back out to straight legs and return to resting position.

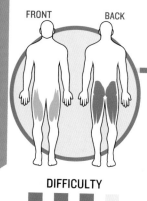

FRONT   BACK

DIFFICULTY

Dumbbell Deadlift

The name says it all—in this exercise, you lift dead weight (in this case, dumbbells) off the floor. Because you hold them separately, you allow your body to move with the weights in a natural way. This exercise targets the major muscles of your lower body—including your glutes, hamstrings, and quads—and gives your core a challenge.

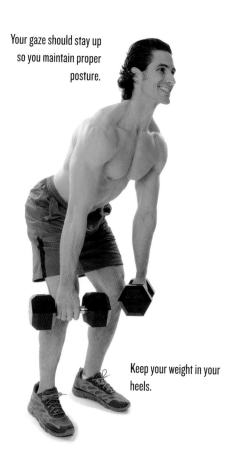

Your gaze should stay up so you maintain proper posture.

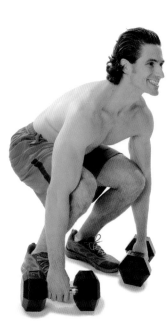

Don't let your knees go past your toes.

Keep your weight in your heels.

1 Stand with your feet shoulder width apart. In a deep forward bend, grab the dumbbells as they rest on the floor.

 Exhale as you stand up and lift the dumbbells off the floor.

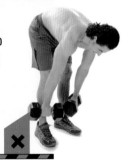
Keep your shoulders relaxed and pulled back.

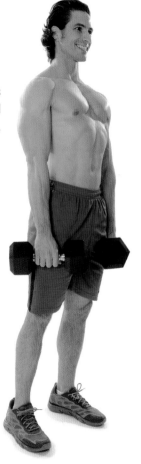

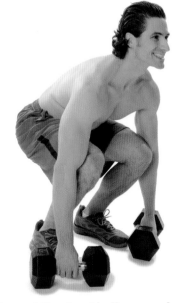

3 Stand completely straight at the top of the deadlift. Allow your hips to extend forward slightly to squeeze your glutes.

4 Control the dumbbells as you lower them back to starting position.

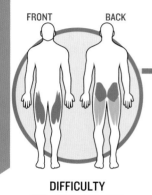

FRONT BACK

Split Squat

The split squat is performed with one leg. This exercise works your quads, glutes, and hamstrings and challenges your balance and core stability.

DIFFICULTY

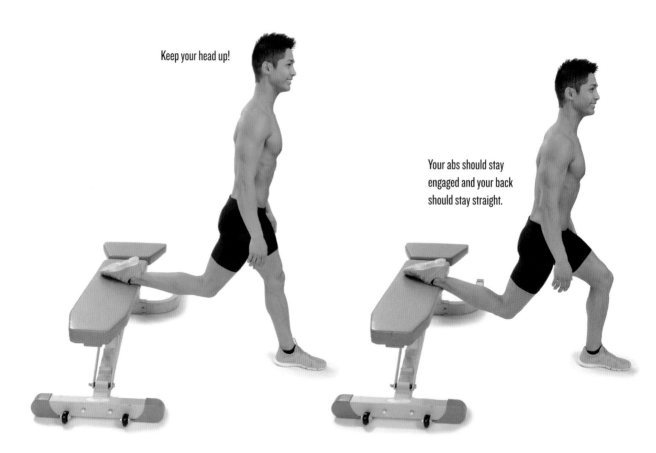

Keep your head up!

Your abs should stay engaged and your back should stay straight.

1 Stand with one foot on the floor and one foot balanced behind you on a bench or step.

2 Inhale and squat down into the lunge.

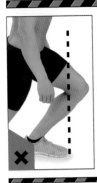

Be Careful!

Make sure to always keep your knees behind your toes. This will protect your knee joints during this advanced exercise.

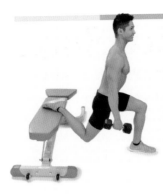

Variation

To progress this exercise and provide an extra challenge for your core, add weight. You can either hold dumbbells down to your sides or a plate or medicine ball at chest level.

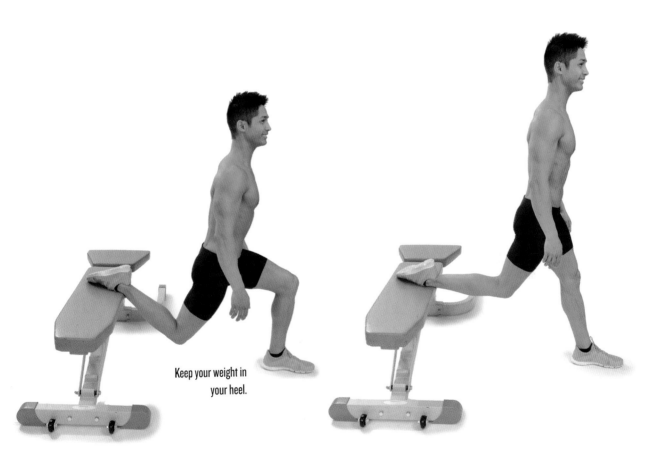

Keep your weight in your heel.

 Pause before your knee reaches the floor. Your legs should be at 90-degree angles.

4 Exhale as you rise back to starting position.

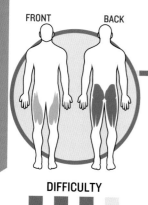

FRONT   BACK

DIFFICULTY

Barbell Deadlift

For this version of the deadlift, you're using a barbell, which requires a great deal of full-body strength. This exercise targets the major muscles of your lower body—including your glutes, hamstrings, and quads—and provides an extra challenge to your core.

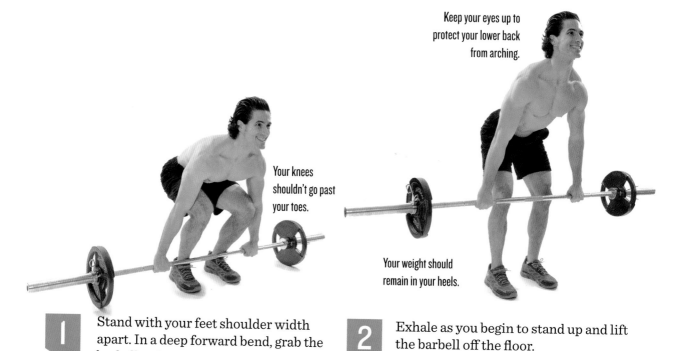

Keep your eyes up to protect your lower back from arching.

Your knees shouldn't go past your toes.

Your weight should remain in your heels.

1 Stand with your feet shoulder width apart. In a deep forward bend, grab the barbell as it rests on the floor.

2 Exhale as you begin to stand up and lift the barbell off the floor.

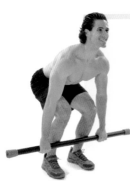

The most important thing to keep in mind when choosing a weight to use is your form. Master the exercise first before adding the barbell and any weight as you progress.

If the Olympic barbell is too heavy for you, feel free to use a lighter fixed barbell for this exercise.

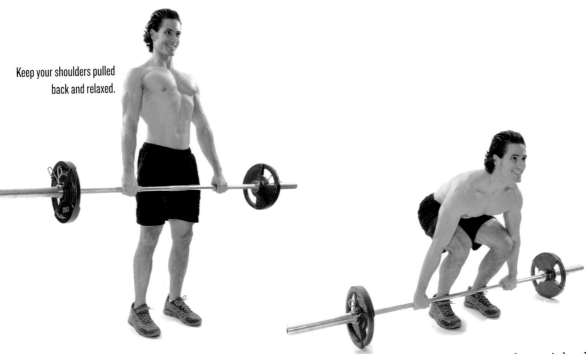

Keep your shoulders pulled back and relaxed.

3 Stand up completely straight, allowing your hips to extend forward slightly.

4 Control the barbell as you lower it back to starting position.

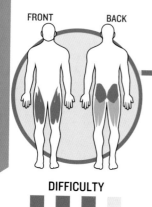

FRONT   BACK

Barbell Squat

This squat progression provides an even greater challenge to your core muscles with the addition of a barbell. It strengthens your abs and lower back along with the major muscles in your lower body.

DIFFICULTY

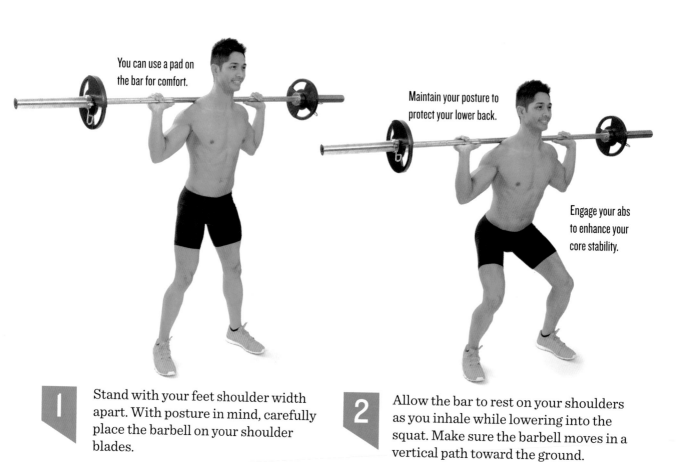

You can use a pad on the bar for comfort.

Maintain your posture to protect your lower back.

Engage your abs to enhance your core stability.

1 Stand with your feet shoulder width apart. With posture in mind, carefully place the barbell on your shoulder blades.

2 Allow the bar to rest on your shoulders as you inhale while lowering into the squat. Make sure the barbell moves in a vertical path toward the ground.

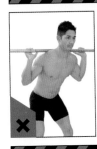

Be Careful!
To avoid injury to your back, don't let it round as you do this exercise. Focus on a spot on the wall as you descend. This will keep your head up and your back nice and straight!

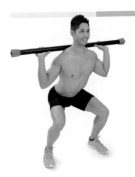

For an easier version of this exercise, try using a fixed barbell instead of an Olympic barbell.

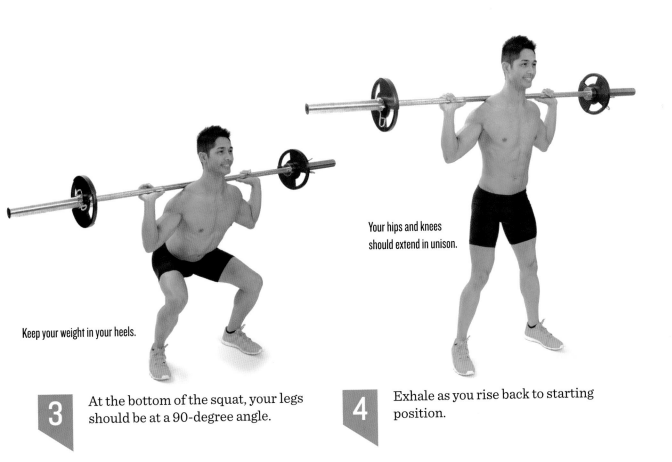

Your hips and knees should extend in unison.

Keep your weight in your heels.

3 At the bottom of the squat, your legs should be at a 90-degree angle.

4 Exhale as you rise back to starting position.

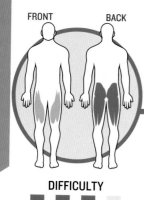

DIFFICULTY

Dumbbell Straight-Leg Deadlift

This exercise builds on the balance and strength challenges of the dumbbell deadlift by requiring you to perform it with straight legs. It targets the major muscles of your lower body, including your glutes, hamstrings, and quads.

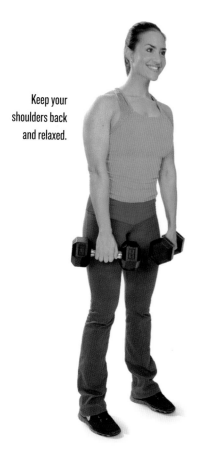

Keep your shoulders back and relaxed.

Your legs should stay still during the entire exercise.

Keep your weight in your heels.

1 Stand with feet shoulder width apart and a slight bend in your knees. The dumbbells should hang comfortably in your hands in front of you.

2 Rock your hips back for a slight pelvic tilt. Inhale as you lower the dumbbells.

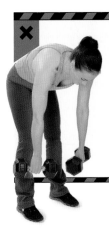

Be Careful!
Pay close attention to your lower back. If you feel pain that isn't related to your muscles doing the move, you may be trying to reach too far with your stretch. Also, if your knees are locked out, it's hard to keep proper form for most people and can create unnecessary strain in your back. This doesn't allow your hamstrings and glutes to perform the exercise properly.

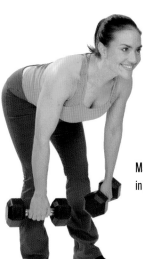

Keep your eyes up to protect your lower back from arching.

Make sure you have a soft bend in your knees.

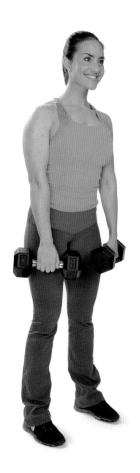

3 Bend at the hips to stretch your hamstrings.

 4 Exhale as you ascend and pull the dumbbells back up to starting position.

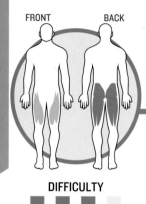

FRONT   BACK

DIFFICULTY

Barbell Straight-Leg Deadlift

Replacing dumbbells with a barbell for the straight-leg deadlift adds a new level of challenge because it requires you to control one fixed weight in front of you. This exercise targets the major muscles of your lower body, including your glutes, hamstrings, and quads.

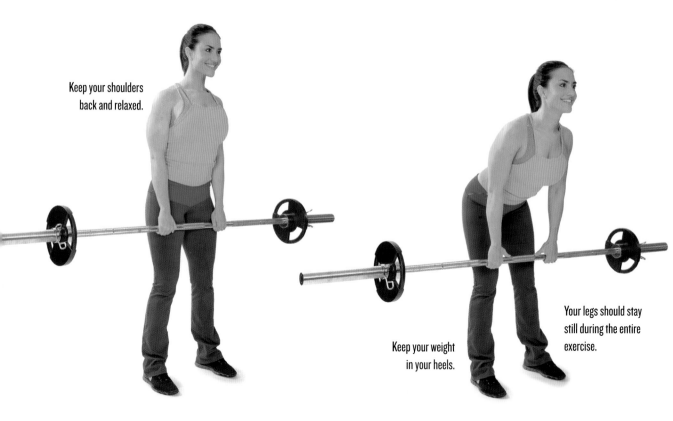

Keep your shoulders back and relaxed.

Keep your weight in your heels.

Your legs should stay still during the entire exercise.

 Stand with feet shoulder width apart and a slight bend in your knees. The barbell should hang comfortably in your hands in front of you.

 Rock your hips back for a slight pelvic tilt. Inhale as you lower the barbell.

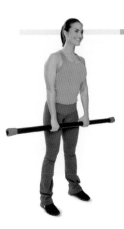

Use a lighter fixed barbell instead of the standard Olympic barbell. This will allow you to perform the exercise with proper form to get the benefits without hurting yourself if the Olympic barbell is too heavy. They come in a wide range of weights to fit every fitness level.

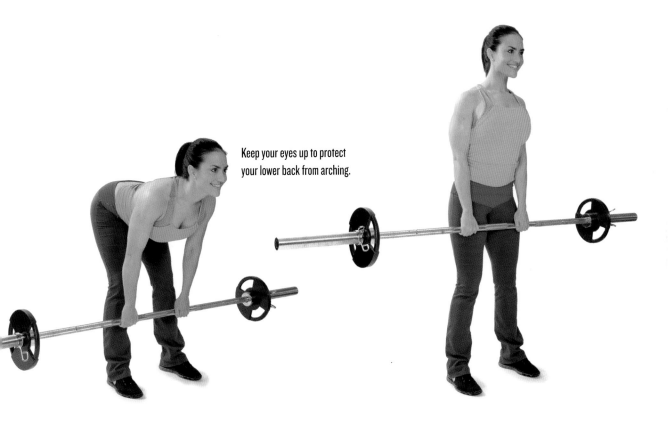

Keep your eyes up to protect your lower back from arching.

3 Bend at the hips to stretch your hamstrings.

4 Exhale as you ascend and pull the barbell back up to starting position.

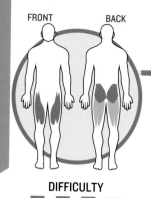

FRONT BACK

DIFFICULTY

Barbell Front Squat

The front squat is almost in a league of its own because having the barbell rest on the front of your shoulders takes double the core strength of a back-weighted squat. Similar to the barbell squat, it strengthens your abs and lower back along with the major muscles in your lower body.

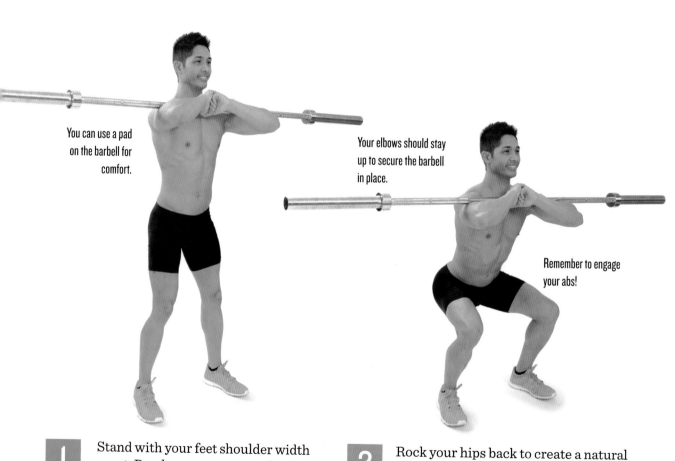

You can use a pad on the barbell for comfort.

Your elbows should stay up to secure the barbell in place.

Remember to engage your abs!

1 Stand with your feet shoulder width apart. Bend your arms out in front of you to allow the barbell to rest on the front of your shoulders.

2 Rock your hips back to create a natural tilt in your pelvis. Inhale as you descend into the squat.

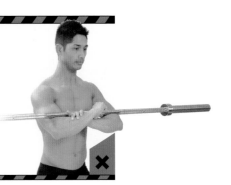

Be Careful!
Don't let the barbell slide down your arms. This can create stress on your upper body and arms that will take away from the squat.

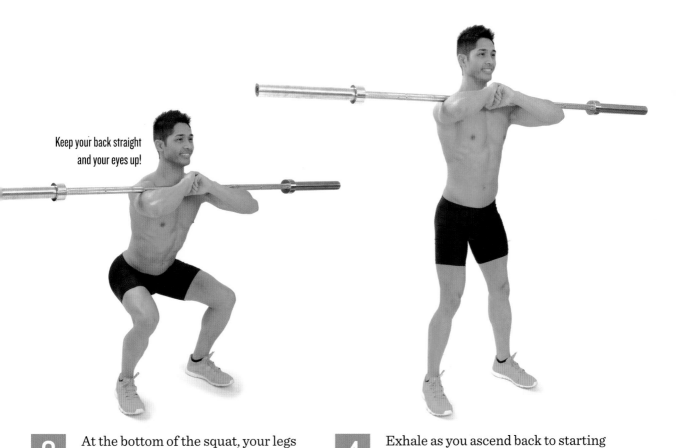

Keep your back straight and your eyes up!

3 At the bottom of the squat, your legs should be at a 90-degree angle.

4 Exhale as you ascend back to starting position.

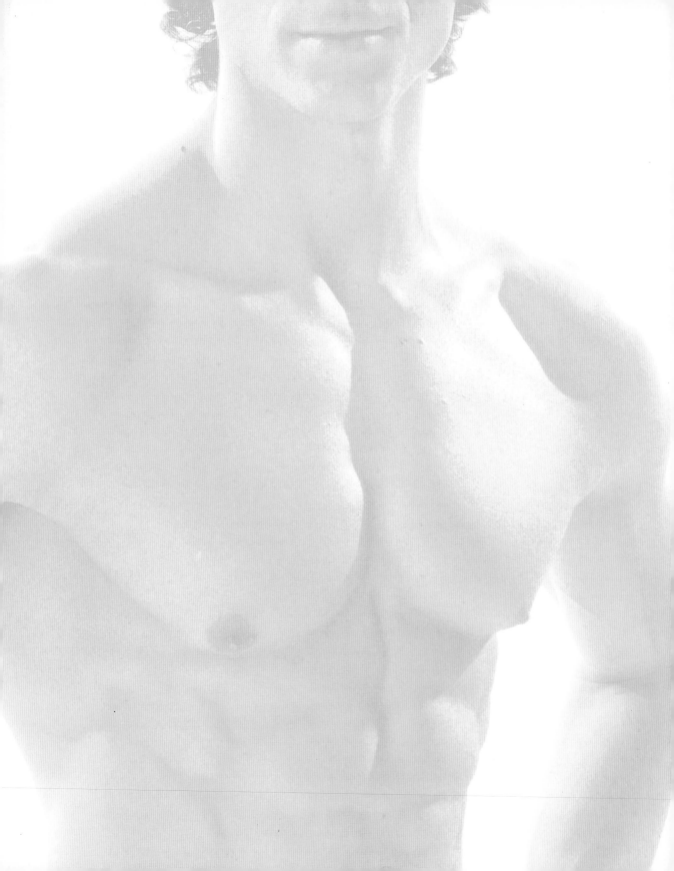

CHEST

(Pecs)

Training the chest isn't just for the buff men and women you see at the beach. Your chest muscles are used in any movements that require lateral arm motion, such as opening a door.

The chest is made up of the pectorals, simply referred to as **pecs.** You use your pecs when you flex your shoulders by pulling your arms forward. When working muscles in your back, your pecs are used to pull your arms down and toward your body. Most chest exercises are also aided by the front deltoids in your shoulders because they are aligned with the pecs.

With some training of the muscles in your chest, you'll better your physique and even improve your posture. You'll also find that completing everyday tasks—like driving your car, washing windows, and even carrying a heavy load of laundry—becomes easier with a strong chest.

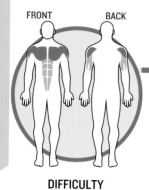

FRONT BACK

Incline Push-Up

The incline push-up is a great way to gain the upper-body strength it takes to perform a standard push-up. By being at an incline, you can still get the same stretch in your pectorals (chest) and front deltoids (shoulders) you do from performing a standard one, but with a little more help from your lower body.

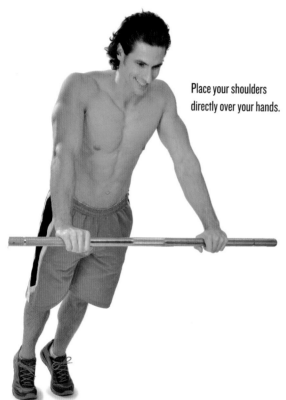

Place your shoulders directly over your hands.

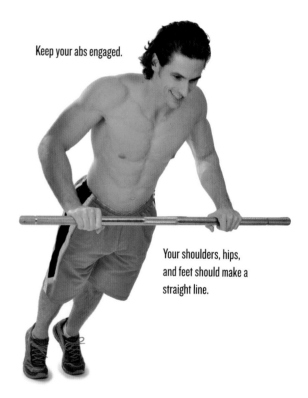

Keep your abs engaged.

Your shoulders, hips, and feet should make a straight line.

1 Set the bar at your desired incline, and hold yourself up off it.

2 Inhale as you lower yourself to the bar.

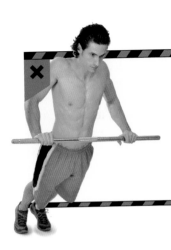

Be Careful!

When performing this exercise, make sure to tilt your hips slightly up to protect your lower back and allow your abs to be engaged during the entire move—don't let your hips drop.

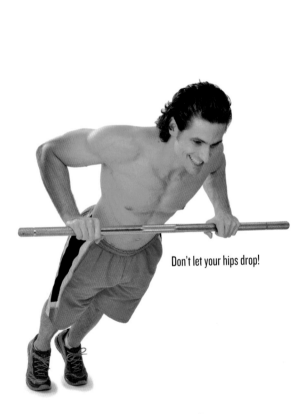

Don't let your hips drop!

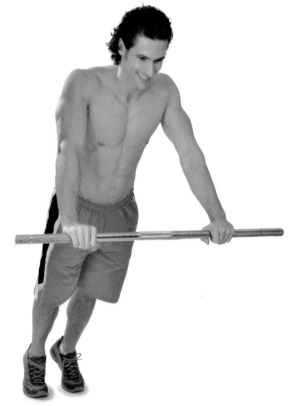

3 At the bottom of the push-up, your elbows should be at a 90-degree angle.

4 Exhale as you ascend back to starting position.

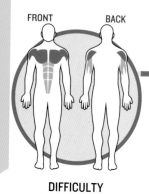

FRONT   BACK

Kneeling Push-Up

The kneeling push-up helps you build up to the standard push-up by protecting your lower back as you build core strength and stability. This exercise primarily works your pectorals (chest) and triceps (arms).

DIFFICULTY

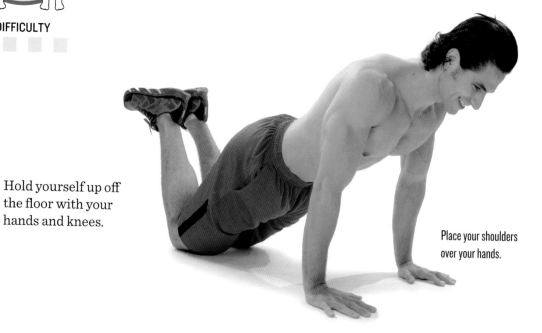

1 Hold yourself up off the floor with your hands and knees.

Place your shoulders over your hands.

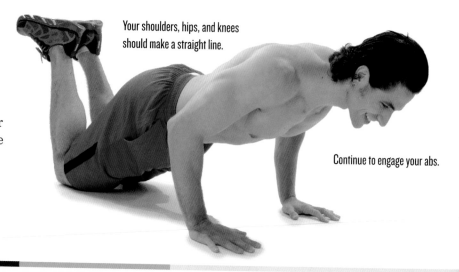

Your shoulders, hips, and knees should make a straight line.

2 Inhale as you lower yourself toward the floor.

Continue to engage your abs.

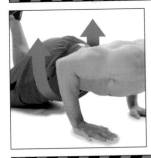

Be Careful!

If you let your hips drop and your arms reach too far away from your body, you could cause injury to your lower back and elbow and shoulder joints. To protect yourself and have proper form, keep your arms directly under your shoulders and your hips slightly tilted up during this push-up.

3 At the bottom of the push-up, your elbows should be at a 90-degree angle.

Keep your hips up!

4 Exhale as you ascend back to starting position.

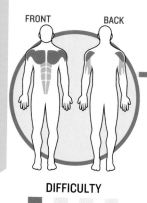

FRONT   BACK

DIFFICULTY

Push-Up

The standard push-up could be considered the single most important exercise for full-body strength and conditioning. Every muscle in your upper body, core, and lower body must be active to perform a push-up with proper form. This exercise targets the muscles in the upper body that do the actual pressing—your pectorals (chest), front deltoids (shoulders), and triceps (arms).

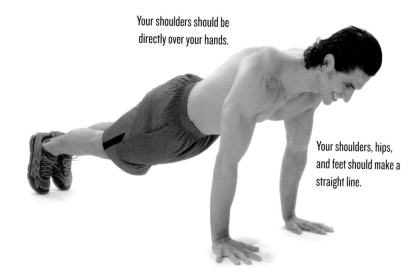

Your shoulders should be directly over your hands.

Your shoulders, hips, and feet should make a straight line.

1 Hold yourself up off the floor with your hands and toes.

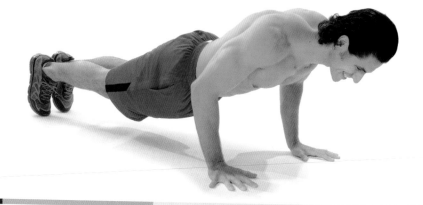

2 Inhale as you lower yourself toward the floor.

Be Careful!

Remember to not let your hips drop during this exercise, as doing so can cause injury. To protect your lower back and keep your abs engaged, your hips should be slightly tilted up.

It's also easy to let your arms reach too far out away from your body, which can cause harm to your elbow and shoulder joints and take the focus off your chest. So be sure to keep your arms directly under your shoulders.

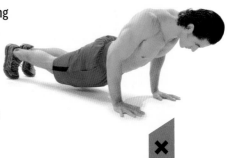

Your abs should remain engaged.

3 At the bottom of the push-up, your elbows should create a 90-degree angle.

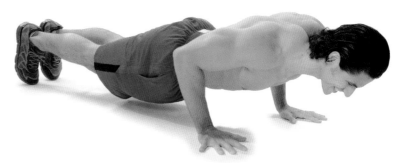

4 Exhale as you ascend back to starting position.

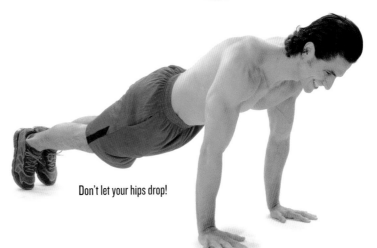

Don't let your hips drop!

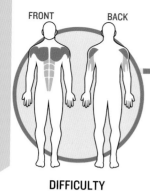

FRONT BACK

DIFFICULTY

Decline Push-Up

To progress the standard push-up, you can do it at a declined angle using a step or bench. This exercise requires extra focus and upper-body strength because the angle takes away the aid your lower body gives you when your feet are on the ground. The decline push-up targets your pecs, front delts, and triceps.

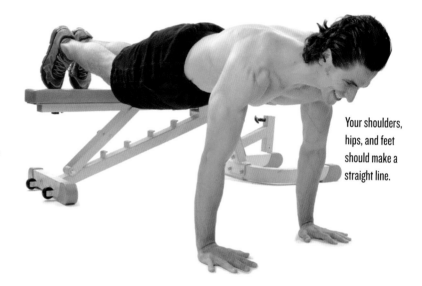

1 Hold yourself up off the floor with your hands, and place your feet above your hips on a step or bench at your desired height.

Your shoulders, hips, and feet should make a straight line.

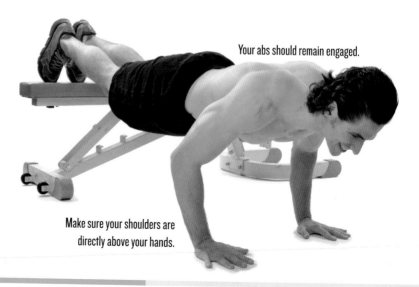

Your abs should remain engaged.

2 Inhale as you lower yourself toward the floor.

Make sure your shoulders are directly above your hands.

Variation

For an additional challenge to the muscles used in this exercise plus their stabilizers, use a stability ball in place of the step or bench. With the ball, your body will have to work harder to stay balanced before you even begin the push-up.

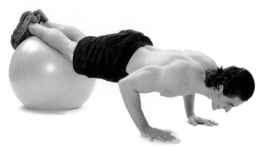

Keep your hips up!

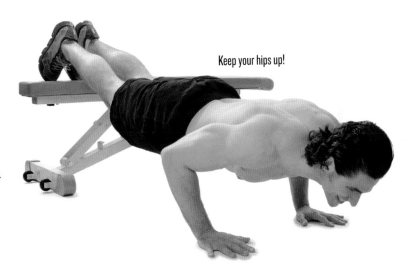

3 At the bottom of the push-up, your elbows should be at a 90-degree angle.

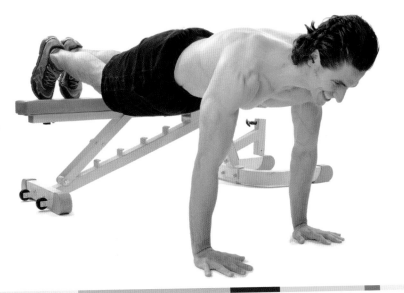

4 Exhale as you ascend back to starting position.

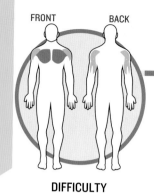
Dumbbell Chest Press

The chest press is a great way to strengthen your pecs, delts, and triceps. Using dumbbells to perform this exercise challenges the stabilizing muscles of your upper body because you're holding weight in each hand separately.

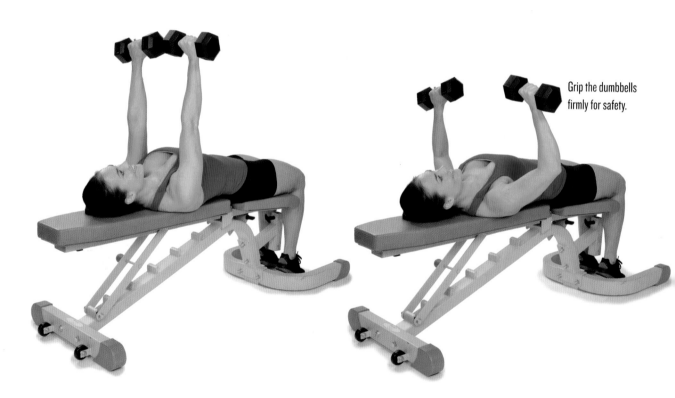

Grip the dumbbells firmly for safety.

1 Lie flat on a bench with your arms naturally extended shoulder width apart to hold the dumbbells.

2 Inhale as you lower the dumbbells to your chest.

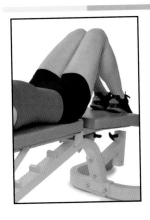

If you feel any stress in your lower back, you can rest your feet on the bench. This will tilt your pelvis in, which will relieve the pressure on your back.

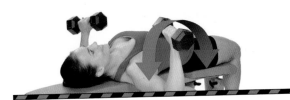

Be Careful!
Don't let the dumbbells fall forward or backward during the press. Doing so can cause unwanted stress to the muscles and joints and possible injury.

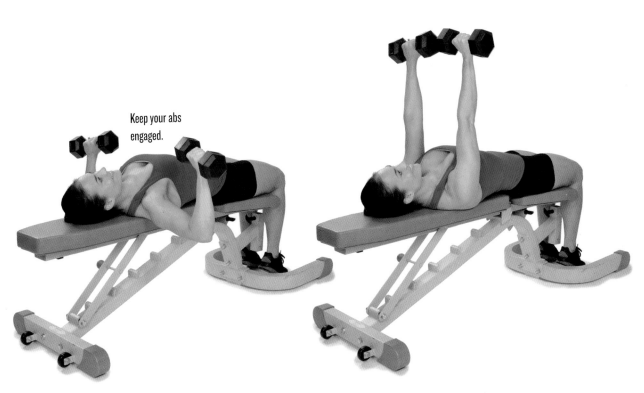

Keep your abs engaged.

3 Allow a stretch in your chest while creating a 90-degree angle with your elbows.

4 Exhale as you press the dumbbells in a straight line back up to starting position.

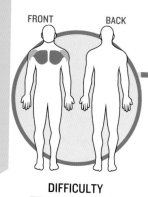

FRONT   BACK

DIFFICULTY

Dumbbell Chest Fly

Similar to the dumbbell chest press, the dumbbell chest fly gives your chest an even greater stretch. You don't use the same amount of weight in this version because your arms are stretched out farther away from your body. This exercise targets your pecs and front delts.

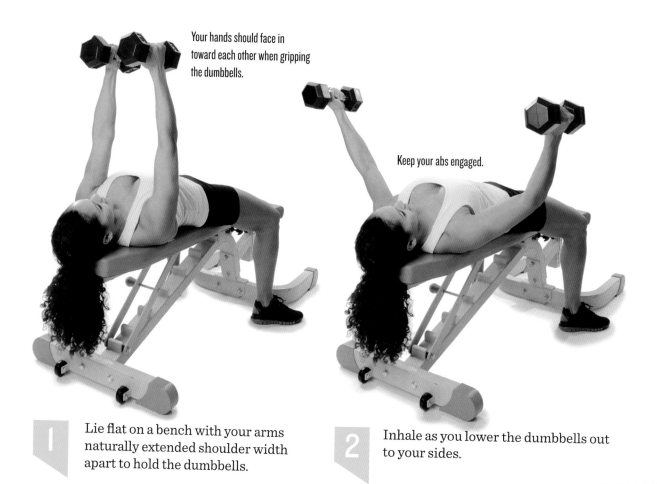

Your hands should face in toward each other when gripping the dumbbells.

Keep your abs engaged.

1 Lie flat on a bench with your arms naturally extended shoulder width apart to hold the dumbbells.

2 Inhale as you lower the dumbbells out to your sides.

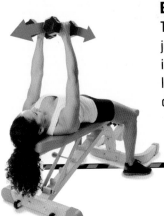

Be Careful!

To protect your elbow joints, keep a slight bend in your arms and avoid letting the dumbbells drop below your elbows.

Variation

To challenge your core and incorporate your lower body, perform this exercise from a stability ball instead of a bench. Make sure to keep your head and shoulders resting on the ball and your feet stable before holding the weights and doing this exercise.

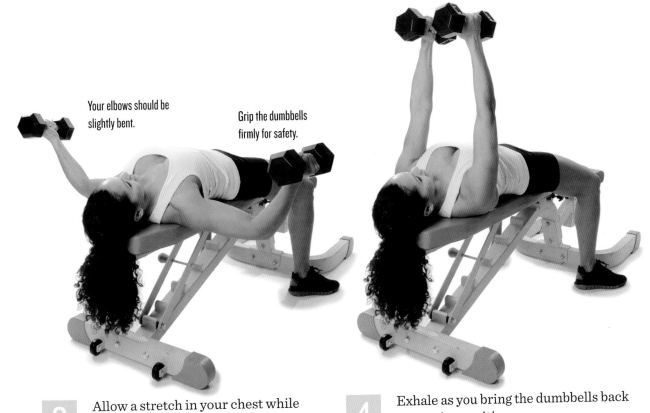

Your elbows should be slightly bent.

Grip the dumbbells firmly for safety.

3 Allow a stretch in your chest while keeping a slight bend in your elbows.

4 Exhale as you bring the dumbbells back to starting position.

Dumbbell Chest Fly

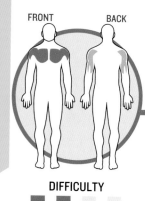

FRONT BACK

CHEST

Incline Dumbbell Chest Press

The dumbbell chest press can be done from an inclined bench to give you a slight angle change. The incline works your shoulder muscles differently than the flat-bench version and can add variety to your chest routine. This exercise strengthens your pecs, delts, and triceps.

DIFFICULTY

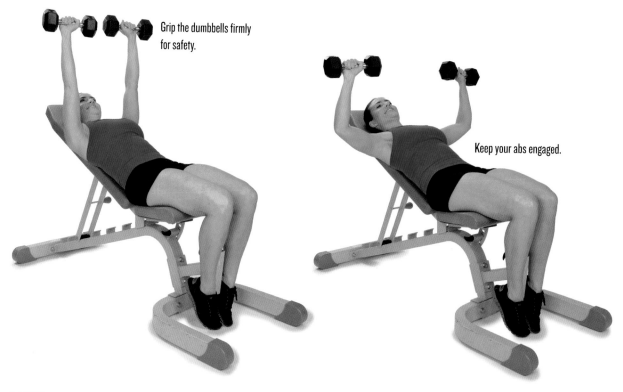

Grip the dumbbells firmly for safety.

Keep your abs engaged.

1 Lie back on an inclined bench with your arms naturally extended shoulder width apart. Hold the dumbbells straight up.

2 Inhale as you lower the dumbbells to your chest.

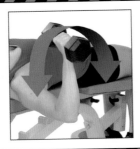

Be Careful!

To avoid unwanted stress to the muscles and joints and even possible injury, don't let the dumbbells fall forward or backward during the press.

Keep your head resting on the bench as your eyes gaze up naturally.

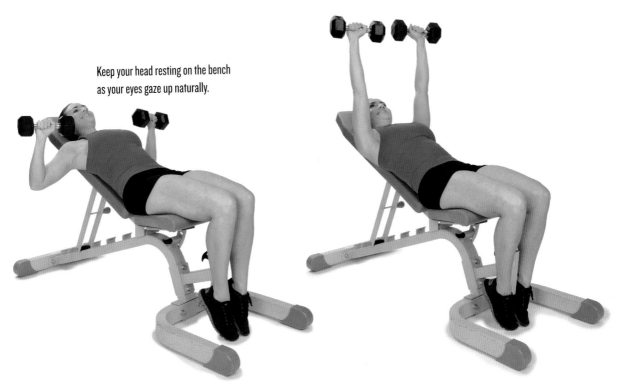

3 Allow a stretch in your chest while creating a 90-degree angle with your elbows.

4 Exhale as you press the dumbbells in a straight line back up to starting position.

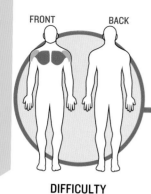

FRONT   BACK

Incline Dumbbell Chest Fly

Performing the dumbbell chest fly from an inclined bench is a nice progression from the flat-bench version. It targets your pecs and front delts, giving the stabilizing muscles in your upper body a challenge.

DIFFICULTY

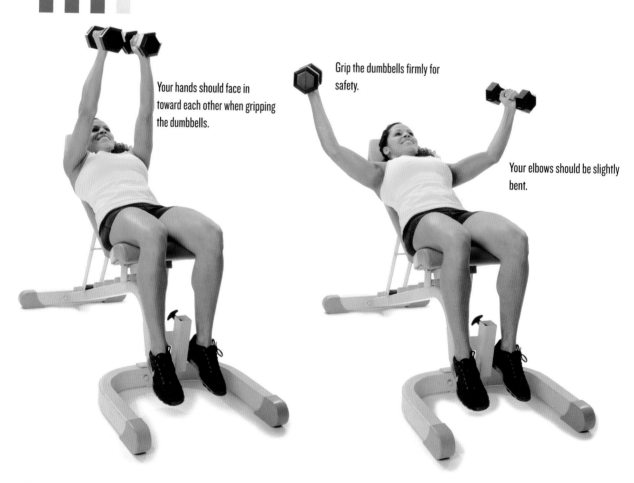

Your hands should face in toward each other when gripping the dumbbells.

Grip the dumbbells firmly for safety.

Your elbows should be slightly bent.

1 Lie back on an inclined bench with your arms naturally extended shoulder width apart to hold the dumbbells.

2 Inhale as you lower the dumbbells out to your sides.

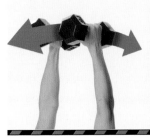

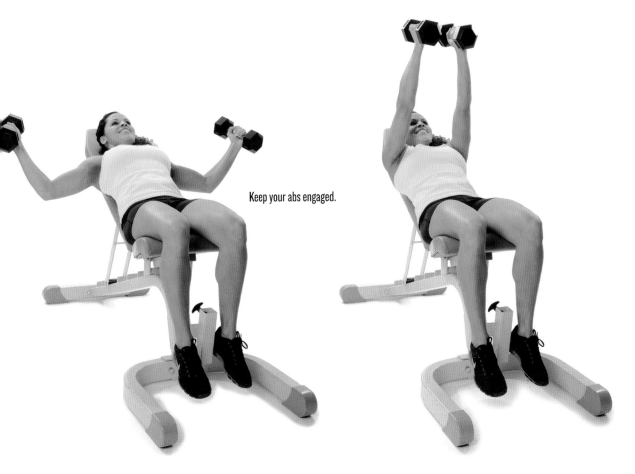

Keep your abs engaged.

3   Allow a stretch in your chest while keeping a slight bend in your elbows.

   Exhale as you bring the dumbbells back to starting position.

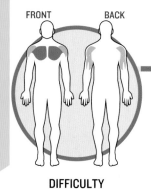

FRONT   BACK

DIFFICULTY

Barbell Chest Press

Once you have become acquainted with the dumbbell version of the chest press, you can increase the difficulty by replacing dumbbells with a barbell. The barbell chest press is a powerful exercise that challenges both your upper-body strength and balance as you hold a long barbell between both hands. This exercise works your pecs, delts, biceps, and triceps.

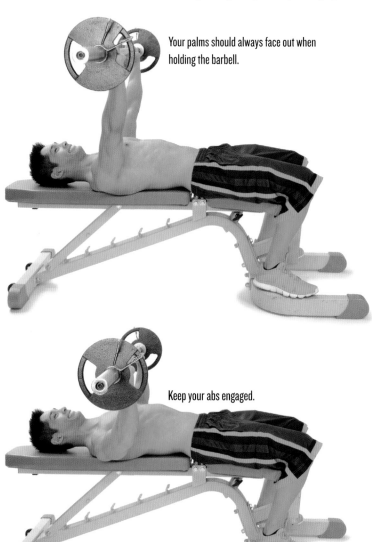

Your palms should always face out when holding the barbell.

Keep your abs engaged.

1 Lie flat on a bench with your arms naturally extended shoulder width apart to hold the barbell.

2 Inhale as you lower the barbell toward your chest.

If you feel the Olympic barbell may be too heavy for you, use a lighter fixed barbell to perform this exercise.

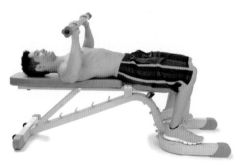

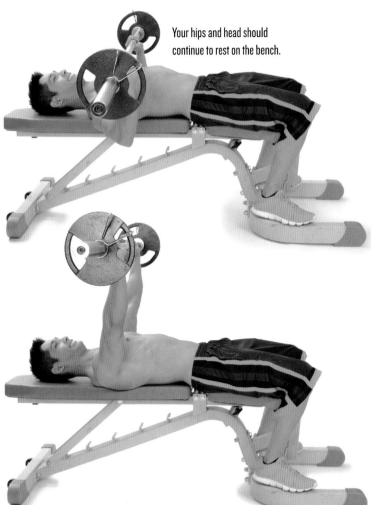

Be Careful!
Don't allow the barbell to fall forward or backward. It takes focus to control the barbell as you not only press it but also keep it moving in a straight line during the entire exercise. Allowing the barbell to fall forward or backward could cause injury to your elbow and shoulder joints and give your upper body an unnecessary workload.

Your hips and head should continue to rest on the bench.

3 Allow a stretch in your chest while creating a 90-degree angle with your elbows.

4 Exhale as you press the barbell back up to starting position.

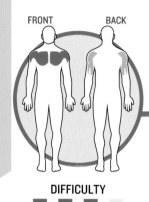

FRONT BACK

Incline Barbell Chest Press

To progress the barbell chest press, you can perform the exercise on an inclined bench. It will incorporate more of your front delts while giving you another option beyond your basic flat-bench routine.

DIFFICULTY

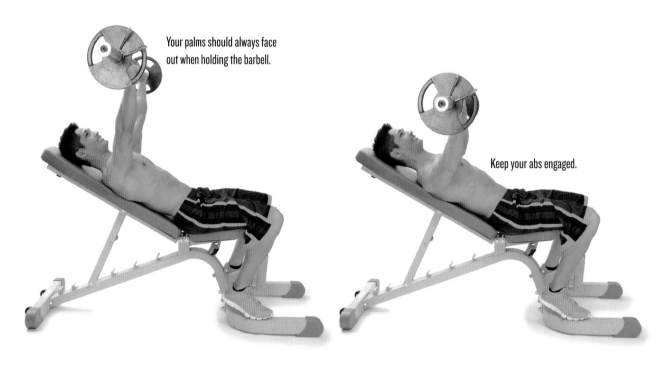

Your palms should always face out when holding the barbell.

Keep your abs engaged.

1 Lie back on an inclined bench with your arms naturally extended shoulder width apart to hold the barbell.

2 Inhale as you lower the barbell toward your chest.

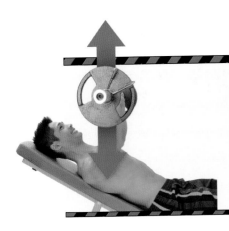

Be Careful!
As in the barbell chest press, focus on controlling the barbell as you press it and keep it moving in a straight line during the exercise—don't allow the barbell to fall forward or backward.

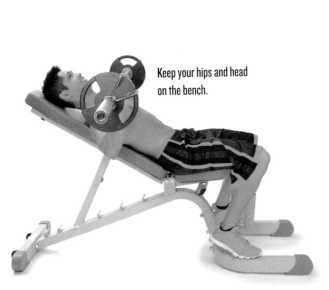

Keep your hips and head on the bench.

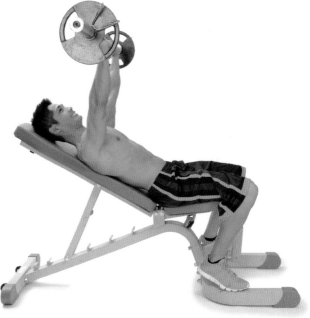

3 Allow a stretch in your chest while creating a 90-degree angle with your elbows.

 4 Exhale as you press the barbell back up to starting position.

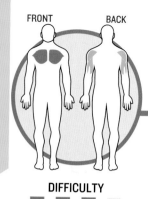
Decline Dumbbell Chest Press

If you'd like to add some variety to your basic flat-bench dumbbell chest press, you can do it on a declined bench. This version of the chest press focuses on your lower pecs.

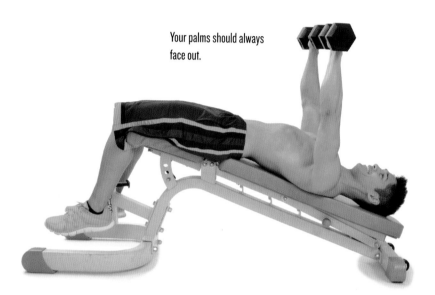

Your palms should always face out.

1 Lie on a declined bench with your arms naturally extended shoulder width apart while holding the dumbbells.

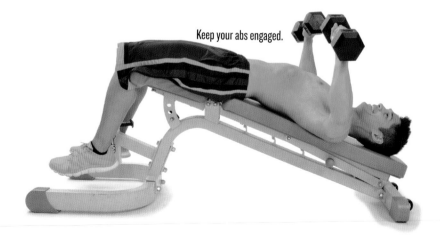

Keep your abs engaged.

2 Inhale as you lower the dumbbells to your chest.

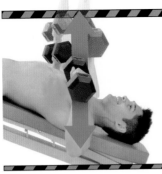

Be Careful!
Don't allow the dumbbells to fall forward or backward. Focus and control the dumbbells so they move in a straight line during the entire exercise.

Keep your head resting on the bench as your eyes gaze up naturally.

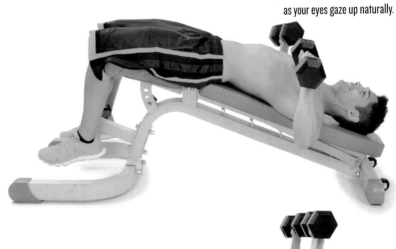

3 Allow a stretch in your chest while creating a 90-degree angle with your elbows.

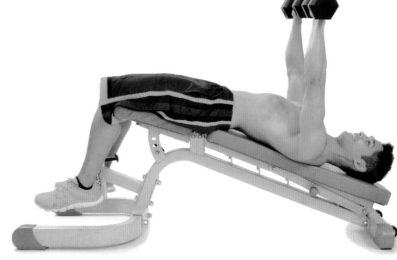

4 Exhale as you press the dumbbells in a straight line back up to starting position.

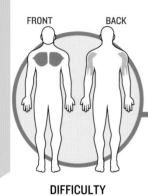

FRONT   BACK

DIFFICULTY

Decline Barbell Chest Press

If you like the incline barbell chest press, you can try replacing the inclined bench with a declined bench. This exercise adds variety to your basic flat-bench routine and focuses on your pecs and triceps.

Your palms should always face out.

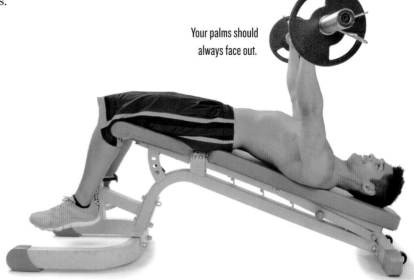

1 Lie back on a declined bench with your arms naturally extended shoulder width apart to hold the barbell.

2 Inhale as you lower the barbell toward your chest.

Keep your abs engaged.

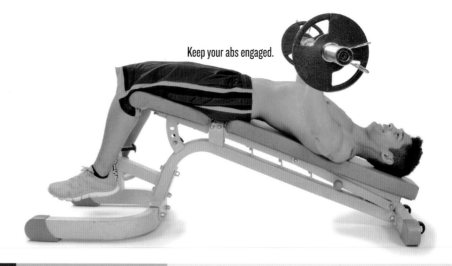

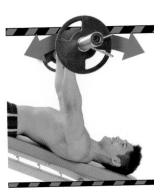

Be Careful!
Remember, don't allow the barbell to fall forward or backward. Focus on controlling the barbell both as you press it and as you keep it moving in a straight line during the entire exercise.

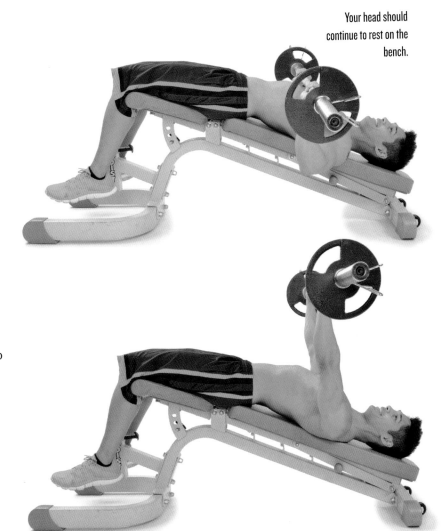

Your head should continue to rest on the bench.

3   At the bottom of the press, allow a stretch in your chest while creating a 90-degree angle with your elbows.

4   Exhale as you press the barbell back up to starting position.

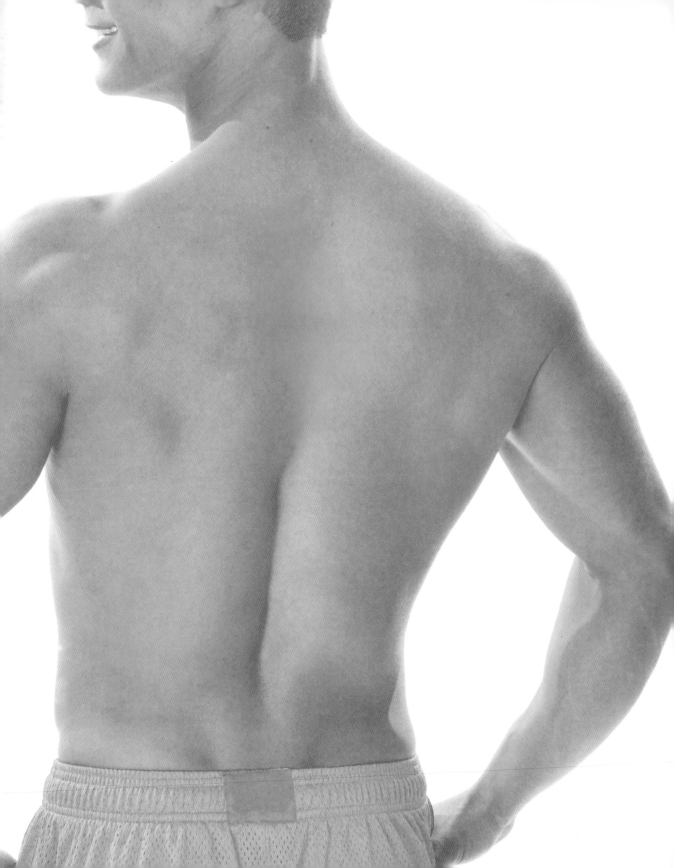

BACK
(Lats and Rhomboids)

Having a "strong backbone" isn't just a saying! Your back is what holds you up and provides stability to the rest of your body, so the benefits of building your back muscles go on and on.

Your back is made up of two muscles: the latissimus dorsi (or **lats**) and the **rhomboids.** While they both must work together to perform major movements, the lats are used more during vertical pulling movements and the rhomboids are used more for horizontal pulling movements.

By building up your back muscles, you'll improve your posture, leading to less back pain. You'll also have stronger lifts for the other muscle groups in the body because you'll be more stable. And having a defined back will make your waist appear slim and small, giving you a "V-body" look—who doesn't desire that?

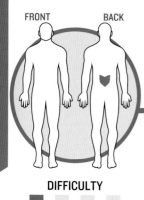

FRONT   BACK

DIFFICULTY

Stability Ball Back Extension

In this exercise, you perform a reverse crunch type of movement to strengthen your core while stabilizing off a stability ball. Strengthening your lower back will help you perform other lower-body exercises, such as squats and deadlifts, with proper form and function. The stability ball back extension targets your spinal erectors (lower back).

1 Lie over a stability ball on your stomach, with your feet on the floor for balance. Inhale as you engage your abs.

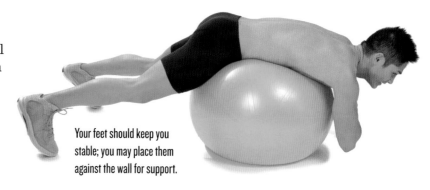

Your feet should keep you stable; you may place them against the wall for support.

Allow your head and eyes to move naturally with your upper body.

2 Exhale as you bring your torso up to squeeze your lower back.

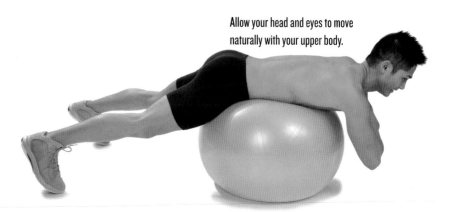

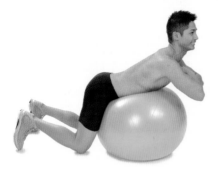

If you feel uncomfortable stability-wise only having your toes touch the floor, you can rest your knees on the floor. Also, keep in mind the size of your stability ball. If your stability ball is too small or too large for your body, your back extension can be completely thrown off.

Keep your abs strong and engaged.

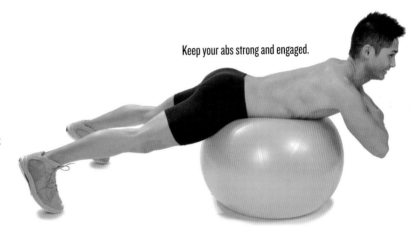

3 Extend up until your shoulders, hips, and knees make a straight line.

The stability ball should remain still.

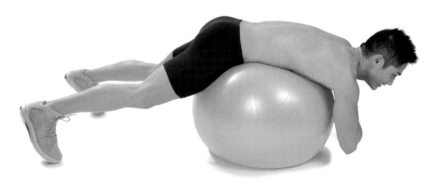

4 Inhale as you return back to starting position.

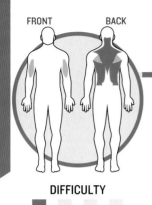

Seated Cable Low Row

The cable low row gives you a base off of which you can build many different kinds of back exercises. This version is performed from a seated position and targets your latissimus dorsi (part of your back), rhomboids (upper back), trapezius (top of your shoulders), and biceps (front of your arm).

DIFFICULTY

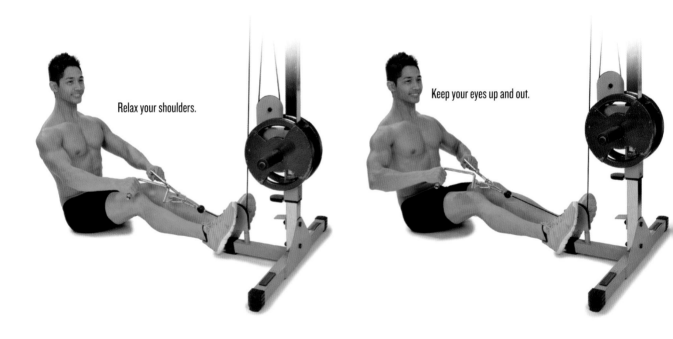

Relax your shoulders.

Keep your eyes up and out.

 Sit with your arms stretched out in front of you. Hold the cable handle naturally.

 Exhale as your pull the cable toward your torso.

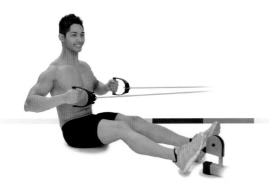

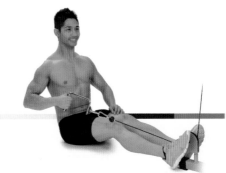

If the cable is too difficult for you starting out, you can use a resistance band and work your way up to the cable.

Variation
Use a single pulley attachment to alternate from side to side. This will provide a bigger stretch to your back and even work your obliques a little more.

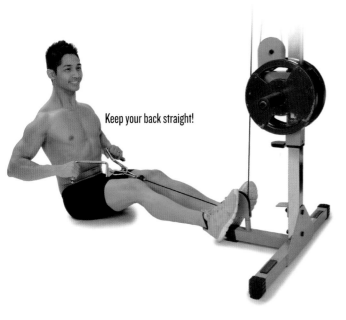

Keep your back straight!

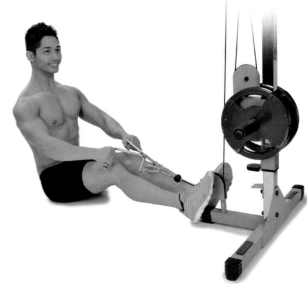

3 Pause to contract your back once your elbows are slightly behind your body.

4 Inhale as you control the cable back to starting position.

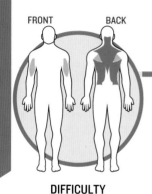

FRONT   BACK

Cable Lat Pulldown

The lat pulldown is a powerful back-strengthening exercise. This exercise targets your latissimus dorsi (part of your back), with help from your rhomboids (upper back), trapezius (top of your shoulders), and biceps (front of your arm).

DIFFICULTY

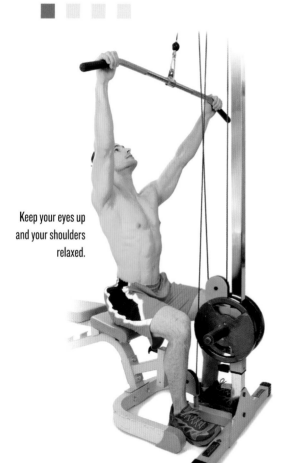

Keep your eyes up and your shoulders relaxed.

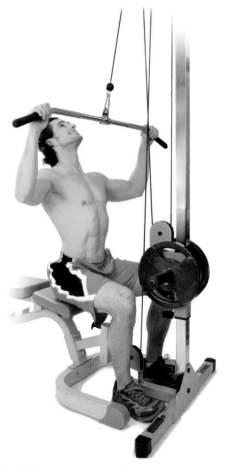

1 Sit with your arms stretched up naturally, just outside of shoulder width. Hold the bar with a prone grip (palms facing forward).

2 Inhale as you stretch to open up your back and abs and begin to pull down the bar.

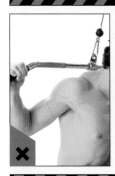

Be Careful!
Don't pull the bar behind your neck. This is a very common mistake that can cause injury.

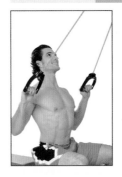

Variation
Use a dual-pulley system to perform this exercise one arm at a time. Alternate from side to side to give your lats a nice stretch and to provide your obliques an extra crunch.

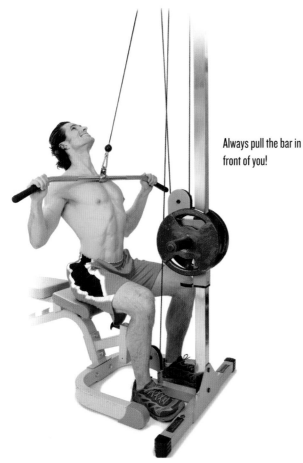

Always pull the bar in front of you!

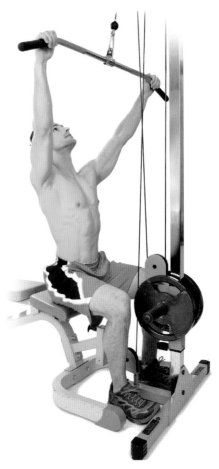

3 Exhale as you pull the bar toward your chest.

4 Inhale as you control the bar back to starting position.

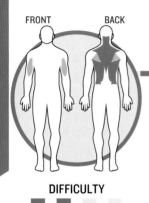

FRONT BACK

Dumbbell T-Bar Row

To perform this exercise, you rest your torso on an inclined bench and row the dumbbells toward you. This exercise targets your rhomboids, with secondary help from your biceps.

DIFFICULTY

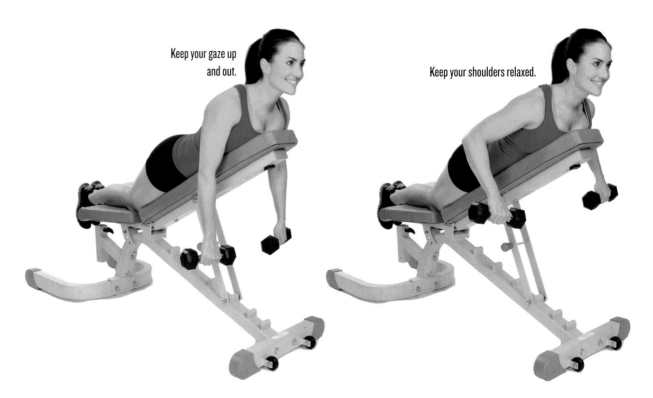

Keep your gaze up and out.

Keep your shoulders relaxed.

1 Rest your torso on the bench and allow the dumbbells to hang down naturally to the floor. Inhale as your back relaxes and stretches out.

2 Exhale as you bend your elbows to raise the dumbbells toward your torso.

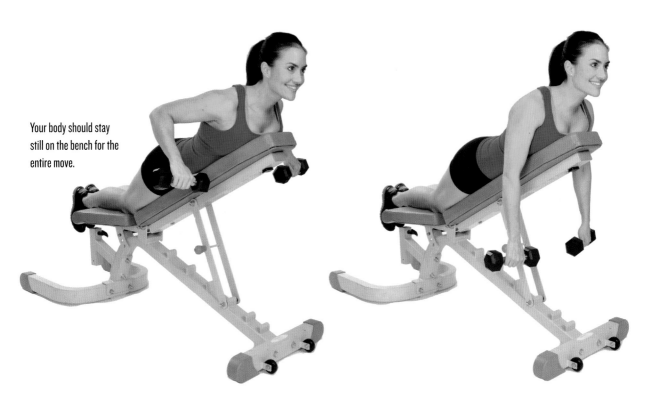

Your body should stay still on the bench for the entire move.

3 At the top of the row, your elbows should be at a 90-degree angle.

4 Inhale as you lower the dumbbells back to starting position.

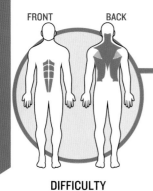

FRONT   BACK

Dumbbell Pullover

The dumbbell pullover is quite the double whammy. It challenges your lats to move the weight without bending your arms and gives your abs a nice stretch.

DIFFICULTY

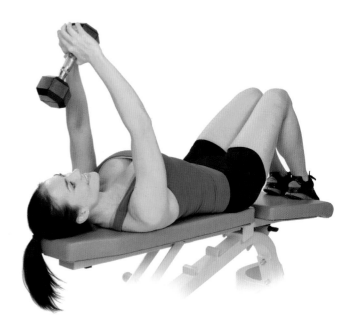

Lie flat on a bench with your arms stretched straight up. Hold the dumbbell vertically at one end of the weight.

It's okay to have a slight bend in your back.

2 Inhale as you lower the dumbbell behind your head.

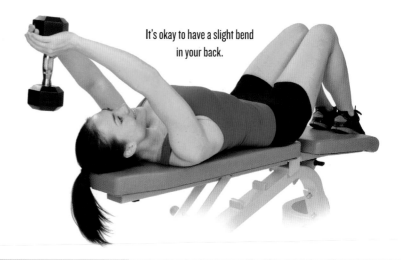

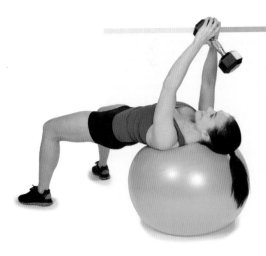

Variation

To give your lower body a challenge, perform this exercise from a stability ball instead of a bench. Make sure your head and shoulders are securely on the ball before holding the weight to perform the pullover.

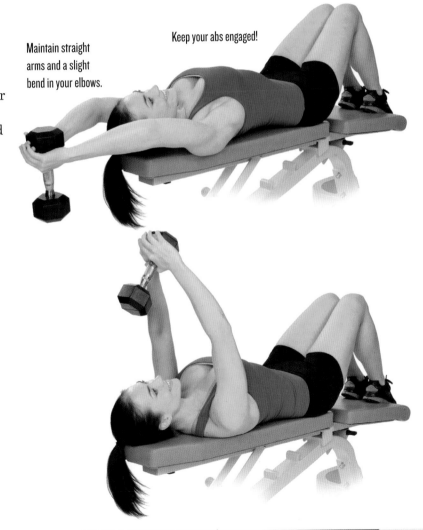

Maintain straight arms and a slight bend in your elbows.

Keep your abs engaged!

3 Pause and stretch your back and abs out once you have fully lowered the dumbbell.

4 Exhale as your bring the dumbbell back to the center of your body.

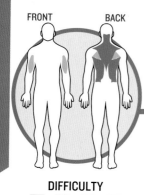

DIFFICULTY

Dumbbell One-Arm Row

The dumbbell one-arm row isolates your back a little more than other versions of the row. This exercise requires your upper body as well as stability in your core and focuses on your lats, rhomboids, and biceps.

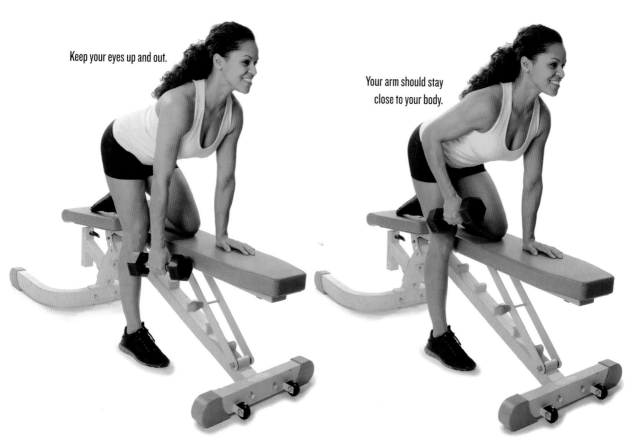

Keep your eyes up and out.

Your arm should stay close to your body.

 1 Support a hand and knee on one side of your body on a bench. Allow the dumbbell to hang down naturally to the floor in your opposite hand.

 2 Exhale as you bend at the elbow to pull the dumbbell toward your torso.

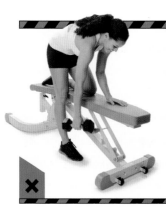

Be Careful!
Make sure you're engaging your back muscles in this exercise by keeping your elbow close to your side. Also, keep your back stretched out long to maintain your form and to avoid letting your lower back round.

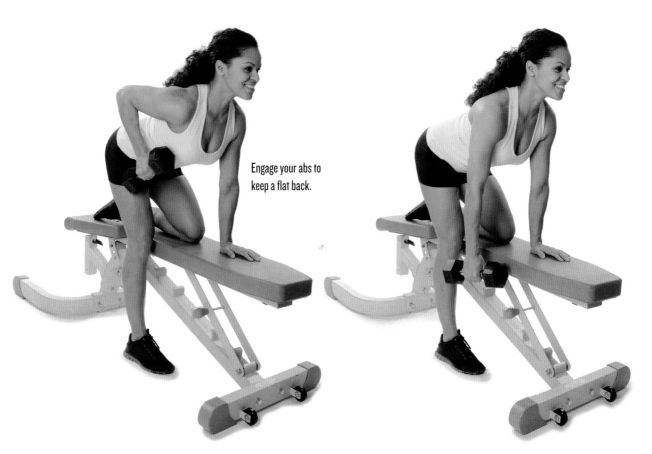

Engage your abs to keep a flat back.

 At the top of the row, your elbow should be at a 90-degree angle.

4 Inhale as you lower the dumbbell back to starting position.

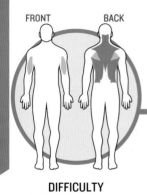

Dumbbell Bent-Over Row

The bent-over row requires most of the muscles in your upper body as well as stability in your lower body. The dumbbell bent-over row targets your lats, traps, rhomboids, and biceps, with a special focus on your traps and rhomboids.

Keep your gaze up and out.

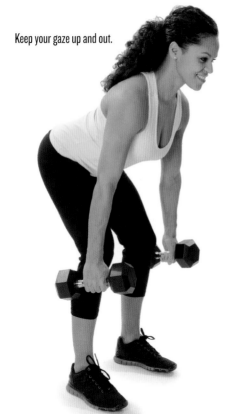

Don't let your shoulders round forward.

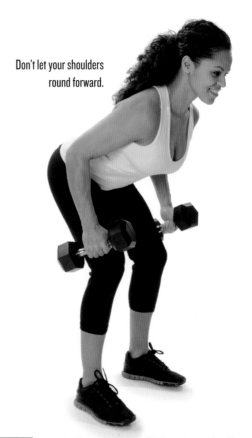

1 Stand with your feet shoulder width apart. With a slight bend in your knees, bend over at the hips and allow the dumbbells to hang down naturally to the floor.

2 Exhale as you pull the dumbbells toward your torso.

Be Careful!

Don't allow the weight of the dumbbells to pull your shoulders forward and create a rounded upper back. Also, be sure you're pulling the dumbbells directly up toward your torso and not hinging your elbows forward like you would during a bicep curl or extending them backward like in a tricep extension.

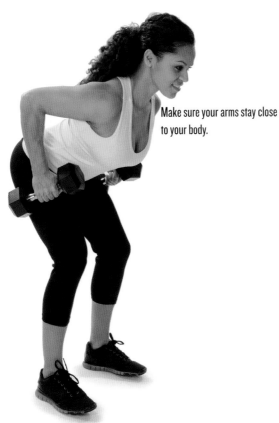

Make sure your arms stay close to your body.

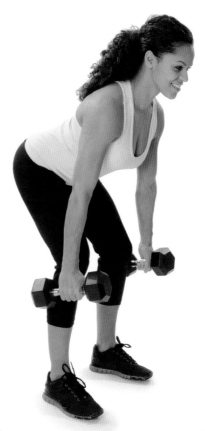

3 Lift the dumbbells until your elbows are at a 90-degree angle.

4 Inhale as you lower the dumbbells back to starting position.

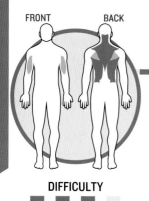

FRONT BACK

DIFFICULTY

Barbell Bent-Over Row

The barbell bent-over row requires the same effort from your full body as in the dumbbell version, with the additional balance challenge of holding a barbell between both your hands. The dumbbell bent-over row targets your lats, traps, rhomboids, and biceps, with a special focus on your traps and rhomboids.

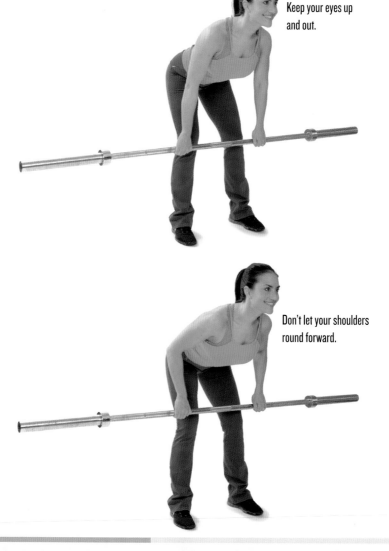

Keep your eyes up and out.

Don't let your shoulders round forward.

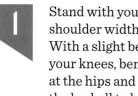

1 Stand with your feet shoulder width apart. With a slight bend in your knees, bend over at the hips and allow the barbell to hang down naturally to the floor.

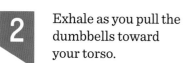

2 Exhale as you pull the dumbbells toward your torso.

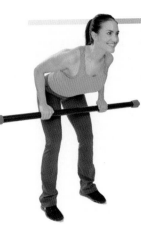

If the Olympic barbell is too heavy for you, use a lighter fixed barbell to perform this movement. It will allow you to keep proper form without your shoulders being pulled forward.

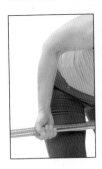

Variation

To get a little extra help from your biceps, switch your grip to palms facing up (supine grip) instead of palms facing down. When using this grip, keep your elbows closer to your sides to protect your elbow joints.

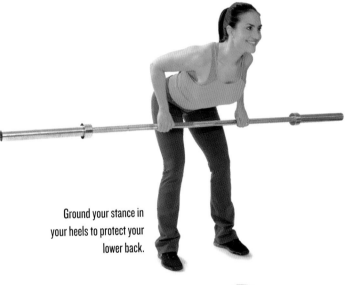

3 At the top of the row, your elbows should be at a 90-degree angle.

Ground your stance in your heels to protect your lower back.

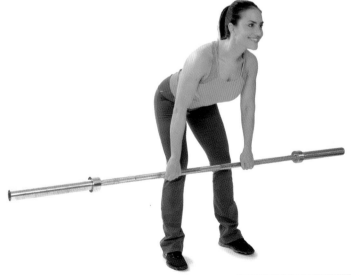

4 Inhale as you lower the barbell back to starting position.

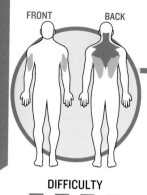

FRONT BACK

Inverted Row

Think of the inverted row as a horizontal pull-up. This advanced exercise for your back targets your rhomboids, lats, and traps and challenges your core by having you keep your body in a straight line.

DIFFICULTY

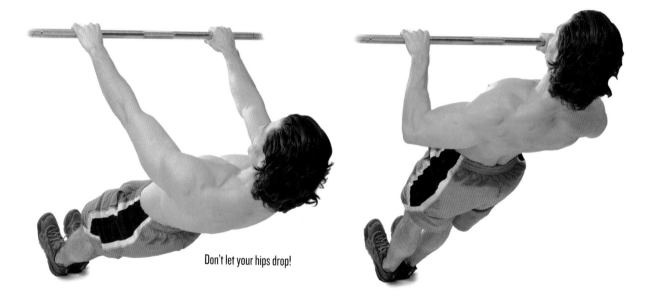

Don't let your hips drop!

1 Hang from the bar with your palms facing down. Rest your feet on the floor.

2 Exhale as you pull your body up toward the bar, keeping your body in a straight line.

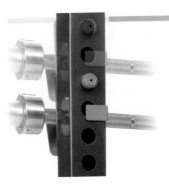

Adjust the height of the bar to your desired level of strength. The higher the bar, the more help you'll have from your legs, making the exercise easier to do.

Your chest should almost touch the bar.

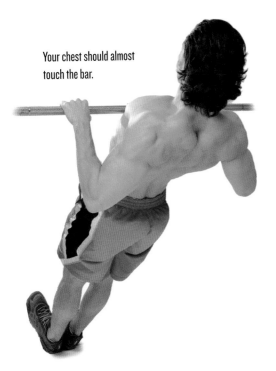

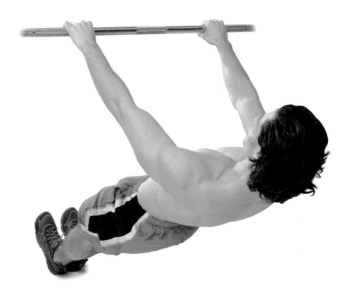

 At the top of the pull, squeeze your shoulder blades together. Your elbows should be at a 90-degree angle.

4 Inhale as your control your body back down to starting position.

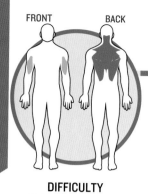

FRONT   BACK

Pull-Up

The pull-up could be the best measure of your upper-body strength. Every muscle in the upper body is used—down to the grip strength in your hands. This exercise targets your lats, with help from your rhomboids, traps, and biceps.

DIFFICULTY

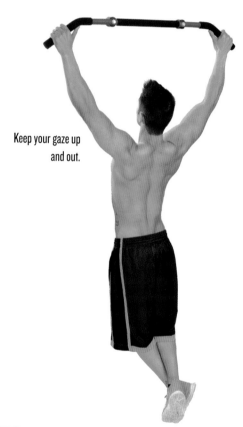

Keep your gaze up and out.

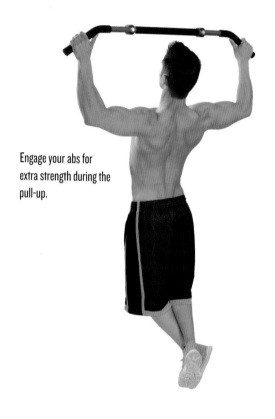

Engage your abs for extra strength during the pull-up.

1 With your arms slightly outside shoulder width apart, hang from the bar using a prone grip. Inhale as you stretch out your back and core muscles.

2 Exhale as your pull your body up toward the bar.

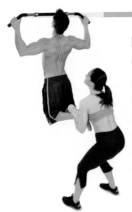

If you aren't to the point where you can do a bodyweight pull-up, have a friend hold your feet or knees to give you the right amount of assistance. This allows you to still perform the exercise while your friend adjusts the amount of help you need.

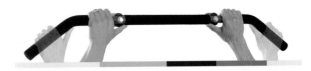

Variation

To make the pull-up easier, simply change to a closer grip. By doing this, the angle in your elbow will be smaller at the top of the pull-up, which will allow your biceps to help more.

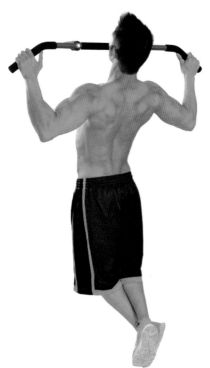

Be sure to stretch out completely at the bottom of your pull-up to get the full range of motion in your back.

3 At the top of the pull-up, your chest should be as close to the pull-up bar as possible.

4 Control your body as you lower back to starting position.

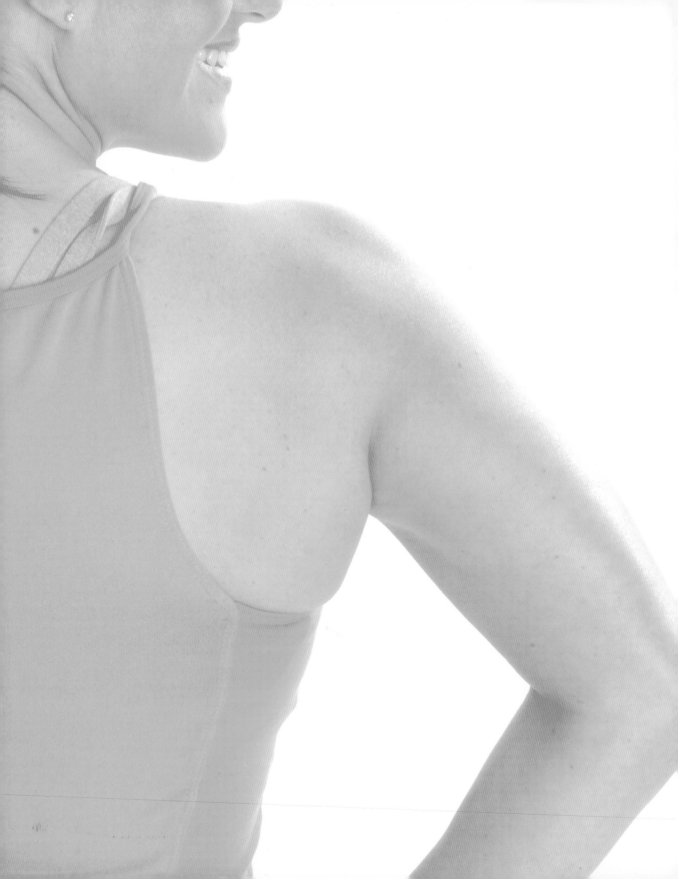

SHOULDERS

(Delts and Traps)

Your shoulders frame your body like your eyebrows frame your face. When you see a rockin' physique, chances are that person has a set of sculpted shoulders! Your shoulders are required to be both mobile (for actions with your hands and arms) and stable (for lifting, pushing, and pulling movements), so building up the muscles in them is important.

The muscles that make up the cap of your shoulder are called deltoids—or **delts** for short—and are made up of the front, medial, and rear delts. Although these muscles are small and act more as "helpers" to the back and chest, they literally carry their share of the work. Ever notice the deep burn from holding a gallon of milk? The stabilizing effort from the delts is very giving and is eager to help throughout day-to-day chores just as much as during a workout. The other muscles that sit between your neck and the delts are the trapezius, or **traps.** The traps are recruited during pulling movements in your shoulders and back.

Having strong shoulders will benefit your daily routine for movements you do multiple times a day, such as reaching for groceries that are above your head at the grocery store and putting away the dishes. Even carrying your computer bag or purse will seem easier with a nice set of conditioned shoulders. And in weight training, having strong shoulders will take away strain from your neck, which often gets a beating.

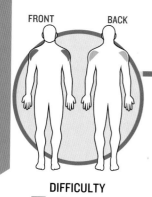

FRONT   BACK

Dumbbell Lateral Raise

The dumbbell lateral raise is a simple exercise that delivers great results. This exercise targets the medial deltoid (middle of your shoulders) through the movement of the dumbbells out away from your body.

DIFFICULTY

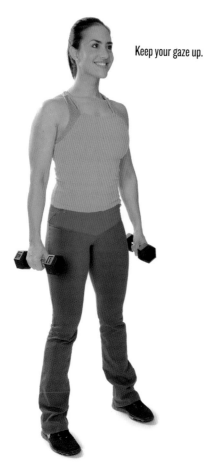

Keep your gaze up.

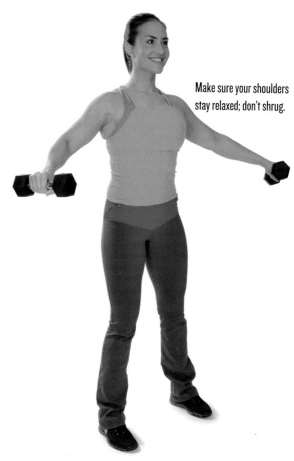

Make sure your shoulders stay relaxed; don't shrug.

1 Stand comfortably with the dumbbells down to your sides.

2 Exhale as you lift the dumbbells out to your sides.

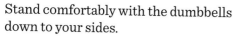

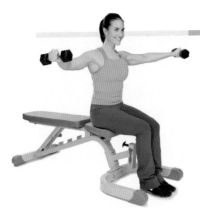

To keep your focus on your shoulders alone, you may perform this exercise from a seated position. Even though your lower body is still during the move, your legs still provide a strong, powerful base to complete the exercise. However, keep in mind that because you're taking away the support from your lower body, you may need to lower the weight you use to keep proper form. Try both versions and do what feels right for your body.

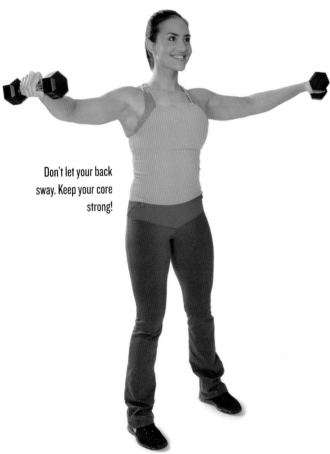

Don't let your back sway. Keep your core strong!

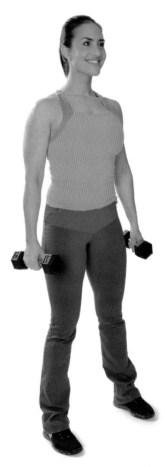

3 Pause once the dumbbells are just beyond parallel to the floor.

4 Inhale as you control the dumbbells back to starting position.

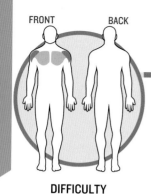

FRONT   BACK

DIFFICULTY

Dumbbell Front Raise

The front raise requires a little more core stability compared to the lateral raise, because you're lifting the dumbbells away from your center of gravity. This exercise targets your front deltoids (front of your shoulders) through the motion of raising the dumbbells up to the front of your body.

Keep your eyes up!

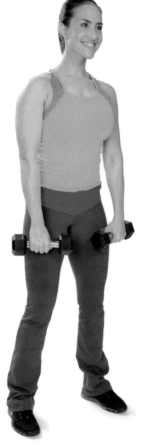

Make sure your shoulders stay relaxed.

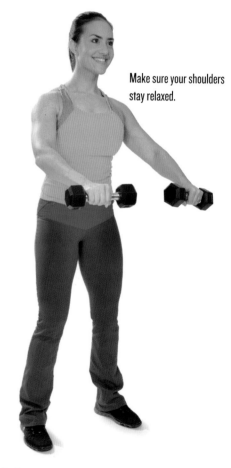

1 Stand comfortably with the dumbbells down to your sides.

2 Exhale as you lift the dumbbells out in front of you.

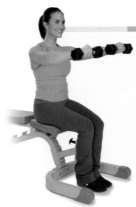

Variation

To change up this exercise, try alternating your front raises separately. This will allow you to focus on one front delt at a time.

You may perform this move from a seated position to allow your focus to be on the shoulders alone. Just know you may need to lower the weight you use to keep proper form in a sitting position.

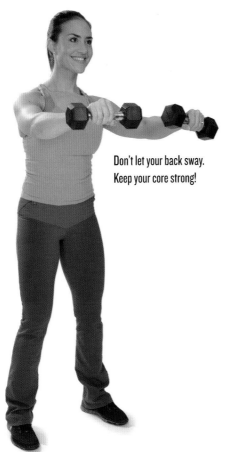

Don't let your back sway. Keep your core strong!

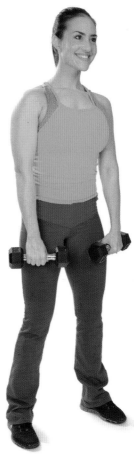

3 Pause once your arms are straight out in front of you.

4 Inhale as you control the dumbbells back to starting position.

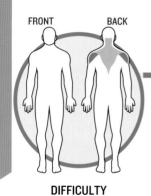

FRONT   BACK

DIFFICULTY

Dumbbell Reverse Fly

The reverse fly is similar to other raises done for your shoulders, except you do this in a bent-over position. This exercise targets your rear deltoids (back of your shoulders).

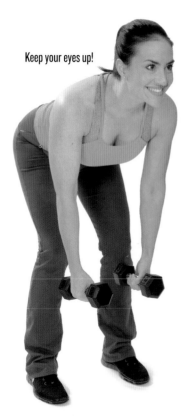

Keep your eyes up!

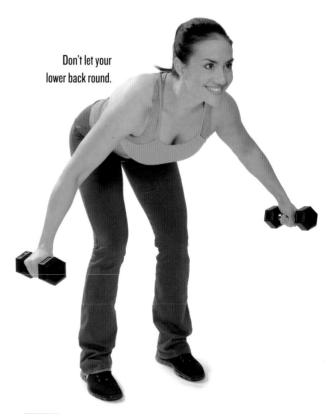

Don't let your lower back round.

1 Stand with your feet shoulder width apart with a slight bend in your knees. Bend over at the hips, and let the dumbbells hang down naturally.

2 Exhale as you lift the dumbbells out to your sides.

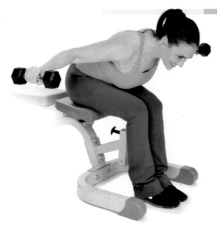

To focus only on your shoulders, you can perform this exercise from a seated position. Even though your lower body is still during the move, your legs still provide a strong, powerful base to complete the exercise. However, because you're taking away the support from your lower body, you may need to lower the weight you use to keep proper form. Try both versions and do what feels right.

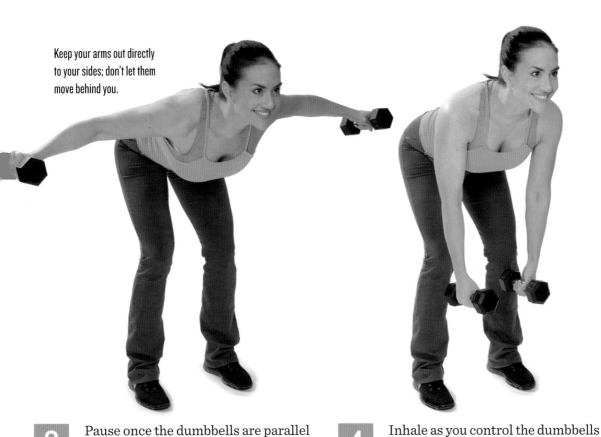

Keep your arms out directly to your sides; don't let them move behind you.

3 Pause once the dumbbells are parallel to the floor.

4 Inhale as you control the dumbbells back to starting position.

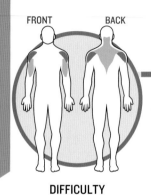

Dumbbell Upright Row

The upright row is a strong exercise to have in your shoulder routine. For this exercise, you must focus on using the front, middle, and rear delts of your shoulder, which ups the level of difficulty compared to the previous dumbbell shoulder exercises.

DIFFICULTY

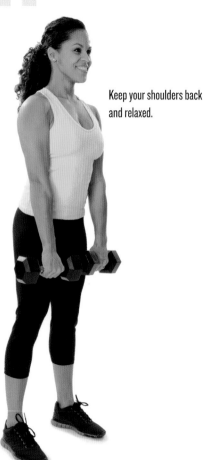

Keep your shoulders back and relaxed.

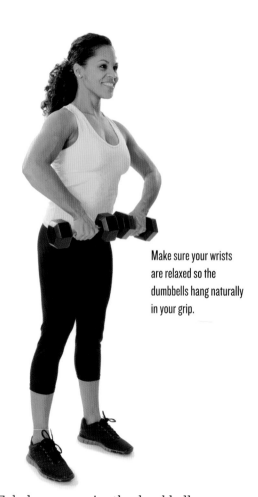

Make sure your wrists are relaxed so the dumbbells hang naturally in your grip.

1 Stand comfortably with the dumbbells down in front of your thighs.

2 Exhale as you raise the dumbbells toward your chest.

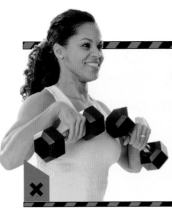

Be Careful!
Be sure to always keep your elbows higher than your wrists and to relax your wrists while holding the dumbbells. If your wrists go above your elbows, you risk injury to both the elbow and wrist joints.

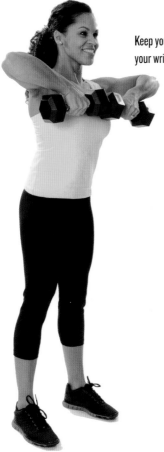

Keep your elbows higher than your wrists.

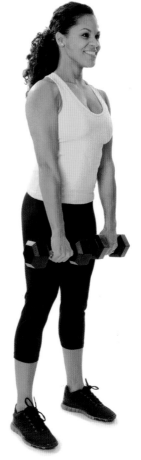

3 Pause once the dumbbells are at chest level.

4 Inhale as you control the dumbbells back to starting position.

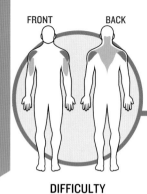

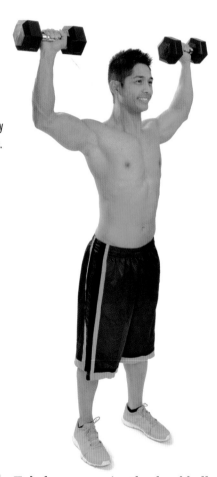

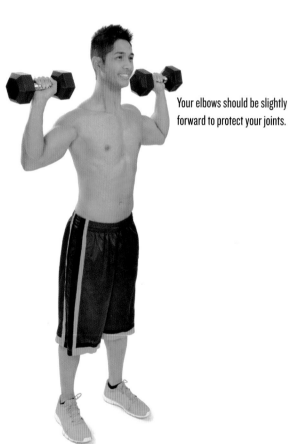

FRONT BACK

DIFFICULTY

Dumbbell Shoulder Press

The shoulder press is an essential exercise to incorporate into your upper-body routine. Using dumbbells in each hand allows your wrists and elbows to move naturally while working your delts, traps, and triceps.

Your elbows should be slightly forward to protect your joints.

1 Stand with your feet shoulder width apart. Hold the dumbbells up at your shoulders.

2 Exhale as you raise the dumbbells straight up.

To allow you to focus on the shoulders alone and not worry about balance while standing, try doing this exercise from a seated position.

Just know that because you're taking away the support from your lower body, you may need to lower the weight you use to keep proper form.

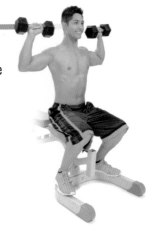

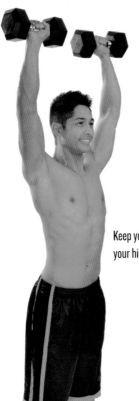

Keep your abs engaged; don't let your hips sway forward.

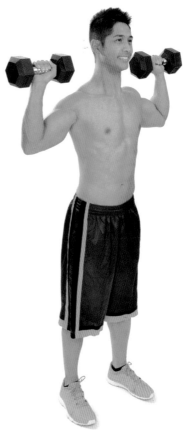

 At the top of the press, straighten your arms.

4 Inhale as you control the dumbbells back to starting position.

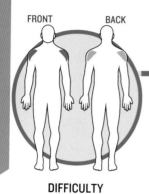

FRONT BACK

Cable Lateral Raise

The cable lateral raise adds a twist to the traditional dumbbell version by replacing the free weights with a cable system to raise the weight away from your body. This exercise targets your medial delt and is usually performed one side at a time.

DIFFICULTY

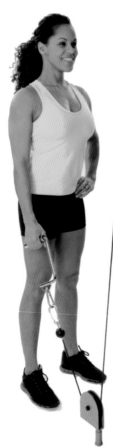

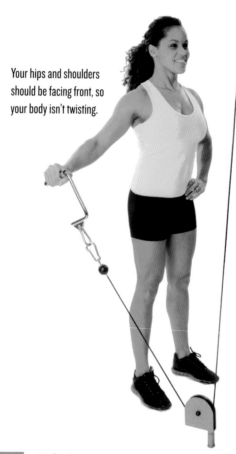

Your hips and shoulders should be facing front, so your body isn't twisting.

1 Stand next to the cable system. Reach across your body with your outside arm to hold the cable handle.

2 Exhale as you raise your arm out to your side.

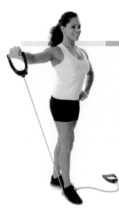

If you feel uncomfortable using the cable, you can use a resistance band instead. This adjustment may feel better on your joints.

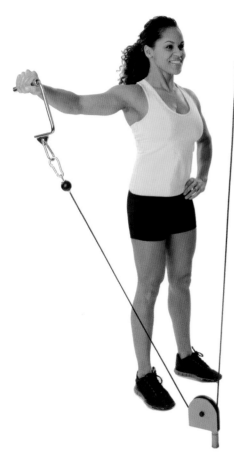

Use controlled movements and keep your abs engaged.

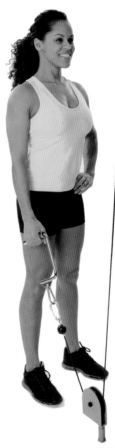

3 Pause once your arm is just slightly past parallel to the floor.

 4 Inhale as you control the cable back to starting position.

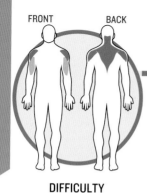

FRONT BACK

SHOULDERS

Cable Face Pull

The cable face pull is like a cable row for the shoulders. The name comes from the movement of pulling the cable toward your face. This exercise targets your rear delts and traps.

DIFFICULTY

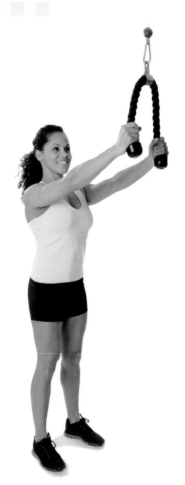

Relax your shoulders.

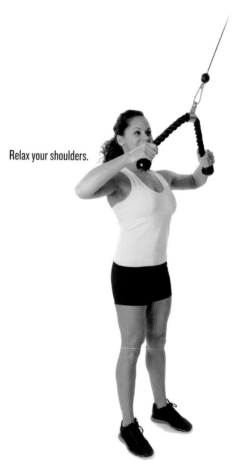

1 Stand with your feet shoulder width apart and your arms out at eye level to grab the cable handle.

2 Exhale as you pull the cable toward your face.

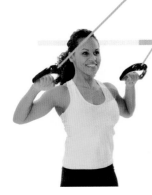

You can use a resistance band instead if you find it difficult to perform this exercise with the cable. After all, it can be hard to relax your shoulders while using them to pull the cable at the same time!

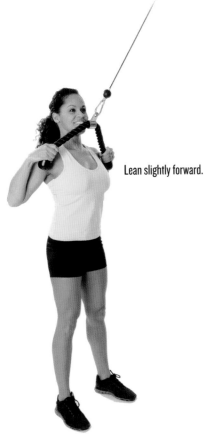

Lean slightly forward.

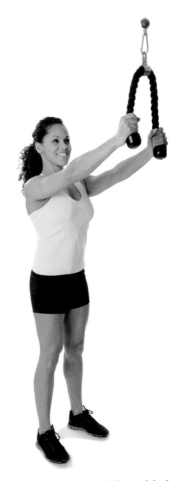

3 Squeeze your shoulder blades together once the cable is near your face.

4 Inhale as you control the cable back to starting position.

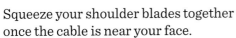

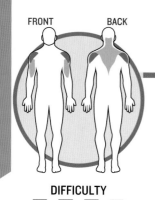

FRONT   BACK

Barbell Upright Row

Using a barbell to perform the upright row adds a challenge to the stabilizers in your shoulders because you must balance holding the barbell between both hands. This exercise focuses on the front, middle, and rear delts of your shoulders.

DIFFICULTY

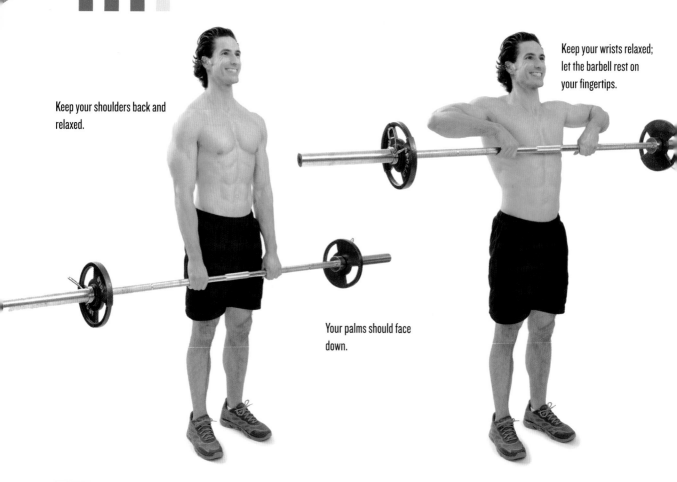

Keep your shoulders back and relaxed.

Keep your wrists relaxed; let the barbell rest on your fingertips.

Your palms should face down.

1 Stand comfortably with the barbell down in front of your thighs. Inhale as you engage your core to stabilize your lower body as your base.

2 Exhale as you pull the barbell toward your chest.

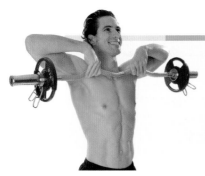

If the Olympic barbell is hard on your wrists, you can use an EZ curl bar for this exercise. The EZ curl bar has grooves that provide more comfort to your wrists than straight barbells.

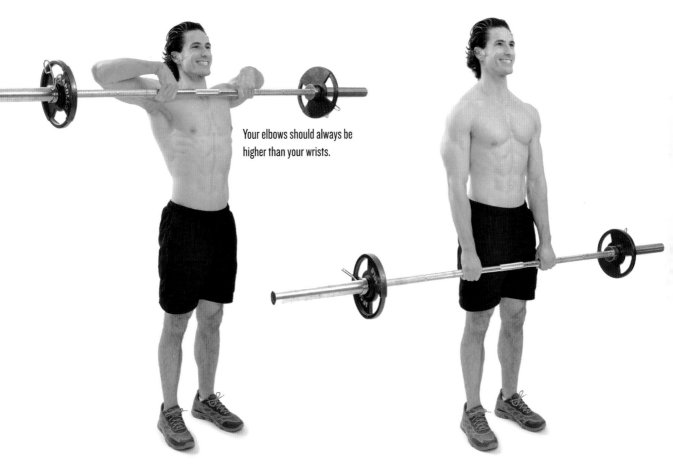

Your elbows should always be higher than your wrists.

3 Bring the barbell to the top of your chest.

4 Inhale as you control the barbell back to starting position.

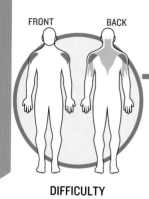

FRONT BACK

Barbell Shoulder Press

The barbell shoulder press requires great stability and core strength in order to balance the long barbell between both hands. This advanced exercise targets your delts, traps, and triceps.

DIFFICULTY

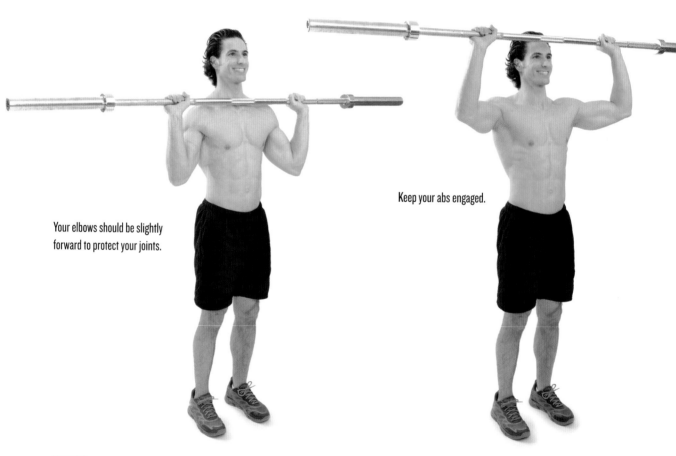

Your elbows should be slightly forward to protect your joints.

Keep your abs engaged.

1 Stand with your feet shoulder width apart. Hold the barbell evenly between both hands at chest level.

2 Exhale as you push the barbell straight up.

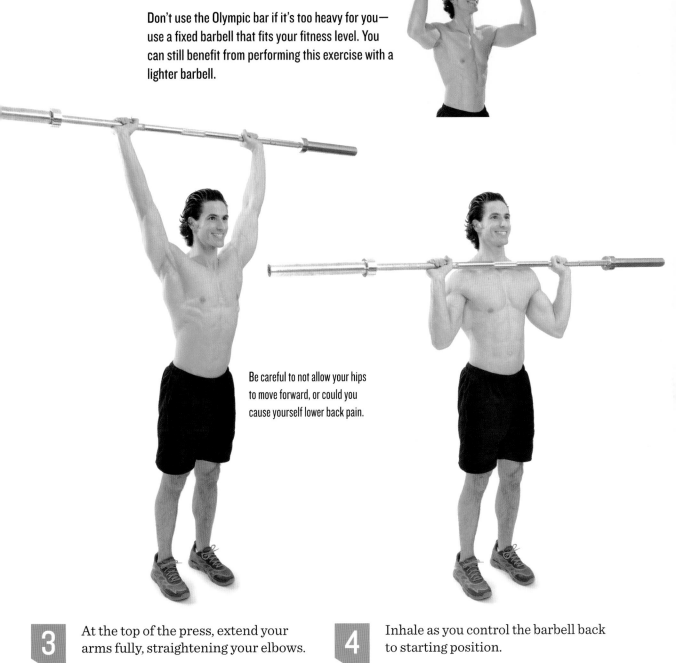

Don't use the Olympic bar if it's too heavy for you—use a fixed barbell that fits your fitness level. You can still benefit from performing this exercise with a lighter barbell.

Be careful to not allow your hips to move forward, or could you cause yourself lower back pain.

3 At the top of the press, extend your arms fully, straightening your elbows.

4 Inhale as you control the barbell back to starting position.

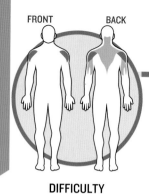

FRONT   BACK

DIFFICULTY

Arnold Press

The Arnold press (named after its creator, Arnold Schwarzenegger) is an advanced version of the dumbbell shoulder press. It is best done in a seated position with smaller, lighter dumbbells. This exercise targets your delts, traps, and triceps, with an extra stretch to your rear delts.

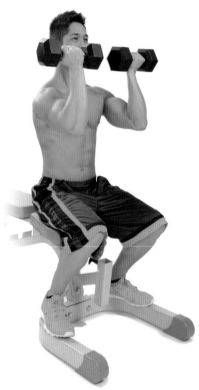

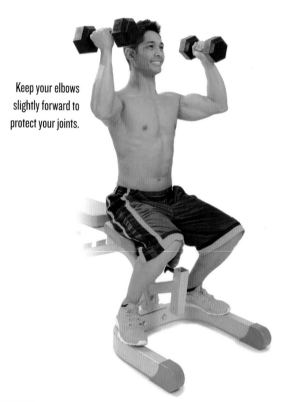

Keep your elbows slightly forward to protect your joints.

1 Bring your elbows together in front of you with your palms facing in.

2 Exhale as you press the dumbbells out to your sides and then press them straight up.

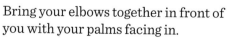

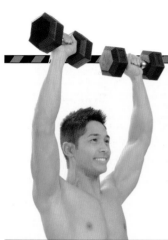

Be Careful!
Be sure to turn your palms out as you press. Keeping them turned in, facing you, can create unwanted stress to your elbows and limit the range of motion in your press.

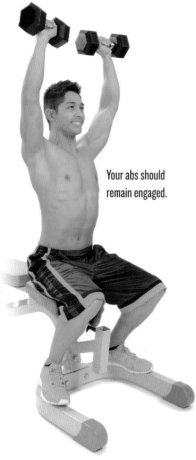

Your abs should remain engaged.

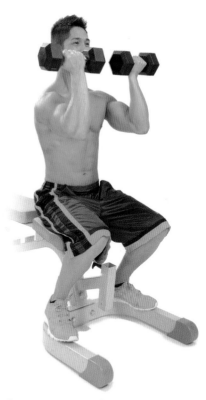

3 Straighten your arms at the top of the press.

4 Inhale as you control the dumbbells back to starting position.

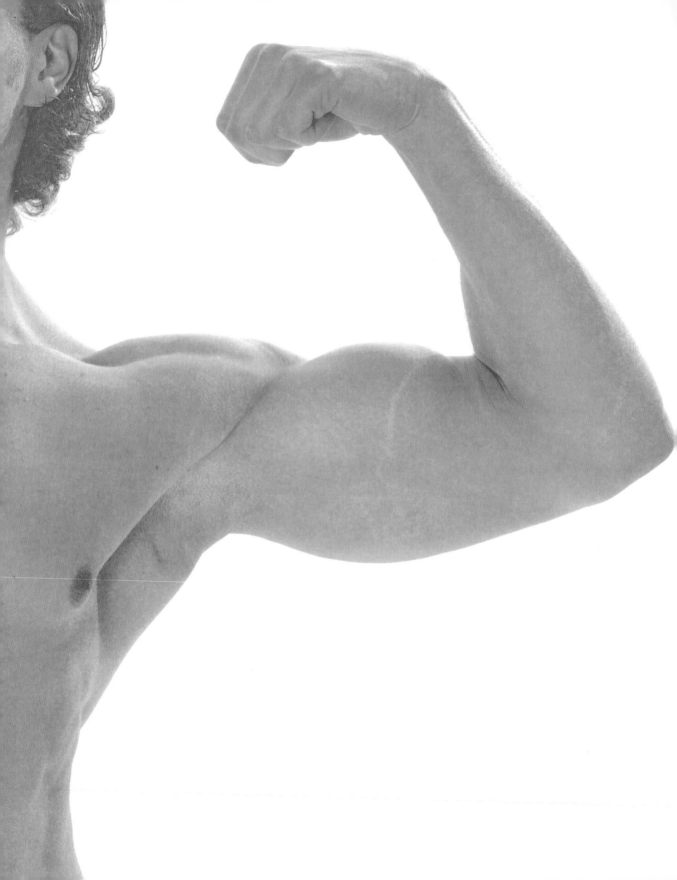

ARMS
(Biceps and Triceps)

Your arms are used in almost every movement you do, such as tying your shoes. However, even with this continual use, your arms can be one of the easiest indicators of your age. And although it may seem like you use your arm muscles a lot, your shoulders and neck usually get the brunt of the work—by elevating your shoulders in a "shrug," you tend to engage them instead of your arm muscles in movements such as pulling up your pants when getting dressed. So strengthening your arms is valuable for both looks and proper function.

Located in the front of your arm, the **biceps** are recruited to help do the pulling during upper-body movements. The **triceps,** in the back of your arm, do the pushing.

By strengthening and stretching your arm muscles, you'll give yourself a long, lean look that helps you avoid the "wave," or underarm flabbiness. You'll also alleviate some of the tension and tightness in your upper back and neck, because your arms will now be more likely to help out.

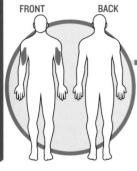

FRONT   BACK

Dumbbell Bicep Curl

The bicep curl seems to be everyone's favorite move because it gives the arms a quick, good pump. This exercise targets your biceps (front of your arm).

DIFFICULTY

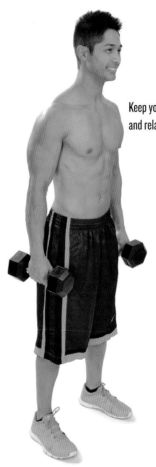

Keep your shoulders back and relaxed.

Your elbows should stay at your sides.

 Stand comfortably with the dumbbells down to your sides.

 Exhale as you bend at your elbows to curl the dumbbells up.

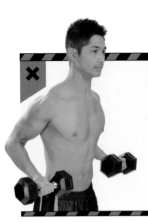

Be Careful!
Don't let your elbows move away from your body. Doing so would take away the work from your biceps and possibly cause injury.

Your palms should face up.

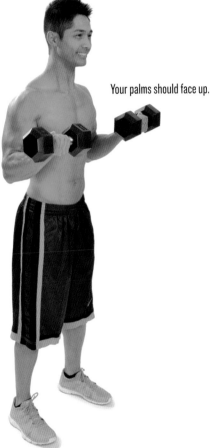

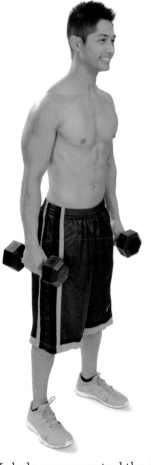

3 Pause once the dumbbells are a little more than halfway up.

4 Inhale as you control the dumbbells back to starting position.

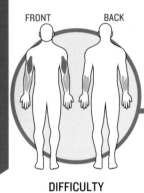

FRONT   BACK

DIFFICULTY

Dumbbell Bicep Hammer Curl

Instead of turning your palms up, the hammer curl uses a neutral grip (palms facing in) for the entire exercise. This slight change in grip makes all the difference and targets your biceps (front of your arms) and abdominals and obliques (torso) while giving your forearms a bit of a challenge.

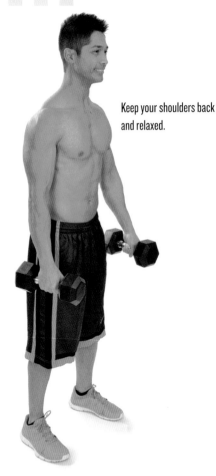

Keep your shoulders back and relaxed.

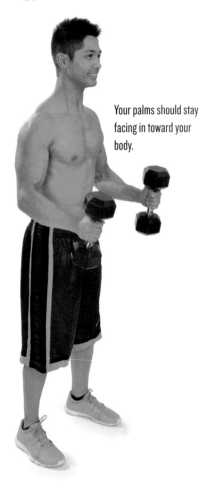

Your palms should stay facing in toward your body.

1 Stand comfortably with the dumbbells down to your sides and your palms in a neutral grip.

2 Exhale as you hinge at the elbow to curl the dumbbells up.

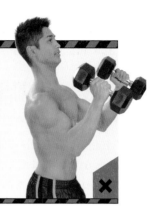

Be Careful!
Don't let your elbows move away from your body. This hinge in the shoulder would take away the work from the biceps and potentially cause injury.

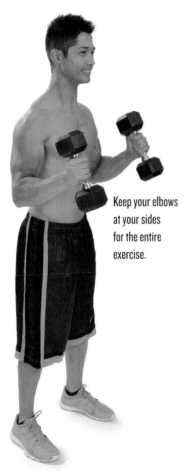

Keep your elbows at your sides for the entire exercise.

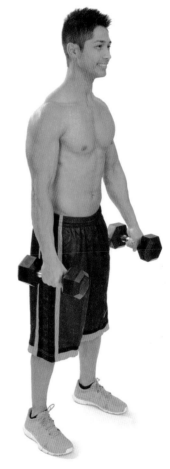

3 Pause slightly past 90 degrees and squeeze your biceps.

4 Inhale as you lower the dumbbells back to starting position.

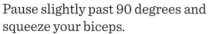

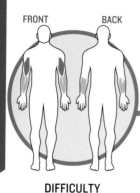

FRONT   BACK

DIFFICULTY

Dumbbell Bicep Reverse Curl

The reverse curl adds a literal twist to the regular curl. Your hands and forearm muscles are challenged because of the prone (palms facing down) grip. This exercise strengthens your biceps (front of your arm) and forearms.

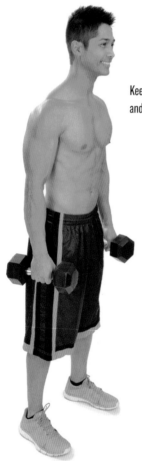

Keep your shoulders back and relaxed.

Your palms should stay facing down.

 Stand comfortably with the dumbbells down to your sides.

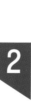 With a prone grip, exhale as you bend your elbows to curl the dumbbells up.

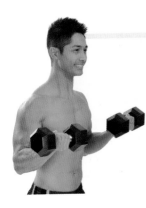

Variation
Try doing a regular curl when bringing the dumbbells up and a reverse curl when bringing them down. You can then switch to reverse curl up and regular curl down.

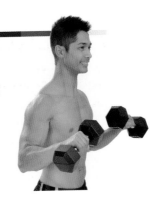

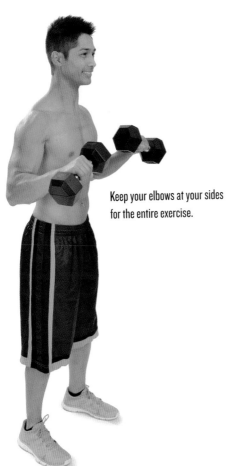

Keep your elbows at your sides for the entire exercise.

3 Squeeze your biceps once the dumbbells are a little more than halfway up.

4 Inhale as you control the dumbbells back to starting position.

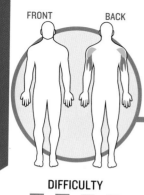

FRONT   BACK

DIFFICULTY

Dumbbell Tricep Kickback

The dumbbell tricep kickback uses the simple hinge at the elbow to go from a bent arm to a straight arm. The bent-over position adds a challenge for your lower body and core. This exercise targets your triceps.

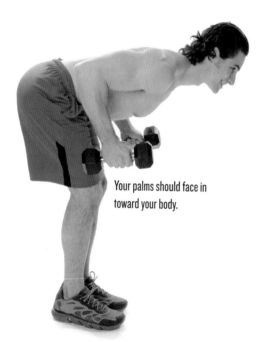

Your palms should face in toward your body.

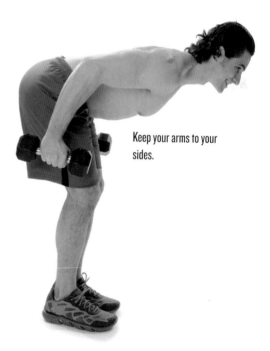

Keep your arms to your sides.

1 Stand with your feet shoulder width apart and your upper body bent over at the hips. Bring your bent arms close to your sides and let the dumbbells hang down naturally. Inhale as you engage your core.

2 Exhale as you extend your arms straight back.

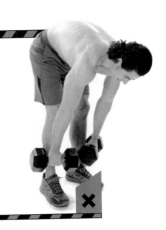

Keep your back straight.

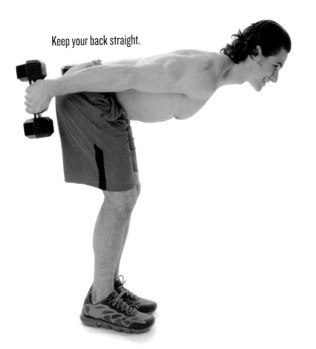

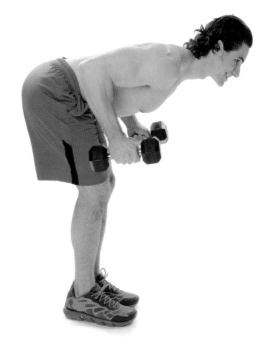

3 Straighten your arms, squeezing your triceps while you do so.

4 Inhale and control the dumbbells back to starting position.

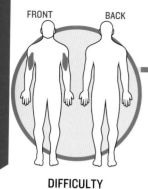

FRONT   BACK

Cable Bicep Curl

Using cables to perform the bicep curl is a nice change from free weights and is done by pulling a rope handle on a cable system. This version targets your biceps and challenges your grip strength in your hands and forearms.

DIFFICULTY

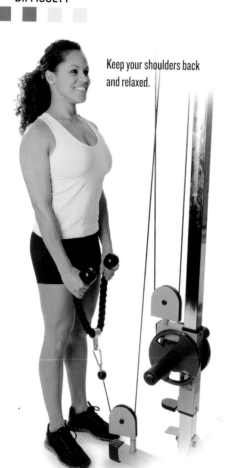

Keep your shoulders back and relaxed.

Your elbows shouldn't leave your sides.

1 Stand with your feet shoulder width apart. Hold the cable handle with a supine (palms facing up) grip.

2 Exhale as you bend your elbows to curl the cable up.

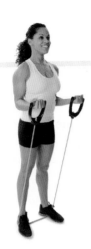

If you're doing this exercise for the first time and the cable seems too heavy, you can use a resistance band to get the same feel of the cables with a little less tension. This version helps you get used to keeping a strong core as you curl the bands.

Your palms should open up to the ceiling.

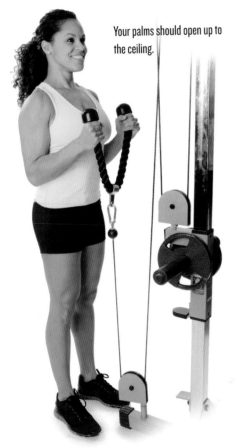

3 Pause once you curl a little more than halfway up.

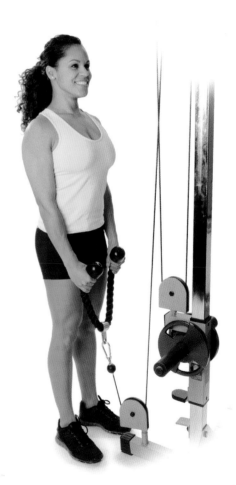

4 Inhale as you control the cable back to starting position.

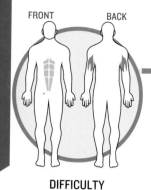

FRONT   BACK

Cable Tricep Pushdown

The cable pushdown is a safe and simple exercise that requires merely going from bent arms to straight arms. This exercise targets your triceps.

DIFFICULTY

Your palms can face each other in starting position.

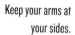

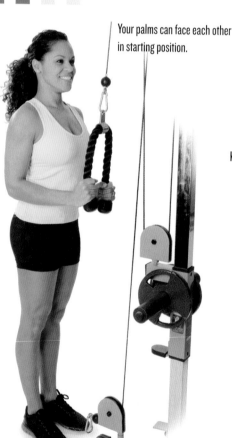

Keep your arms at your sides.

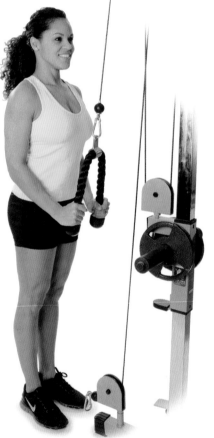

1 Stand with your feet shoulder width apart. With your elbows at a 90-degree angle, hold the cable handle in front of you. Inhale and engage your abs to prepare a strong core.

2 Exhale as your begin to push the cable down toward the floor.

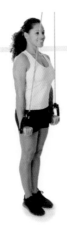

The cable may seem a little heavy if you have never done the move before. Try using a resistance band to perform an easier version of the pushdowns. This will give you the same movement with less tension on your elbow joints.

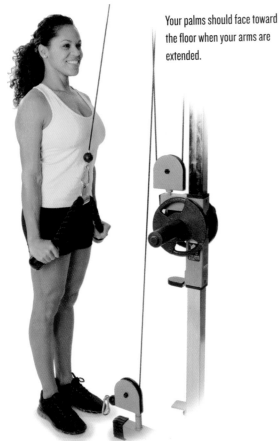

Your palms should face toward the floor when your arms are extended.

3 Pause once your arms are extended straight down.

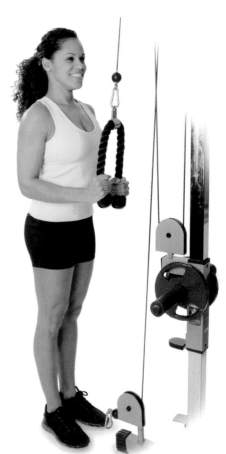

4 Inhale as you control the cable back to starting position.

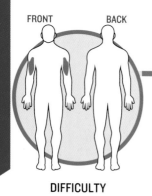

FRONT   BACK

DIFFICULTY

Barbell Bicep Curl

Using a barbell to perform the bicep curl adds the challenge of balancing the barbell between both hands and stabilizing your core as the weight hangs down in front of you. This exercise targets your biceps.

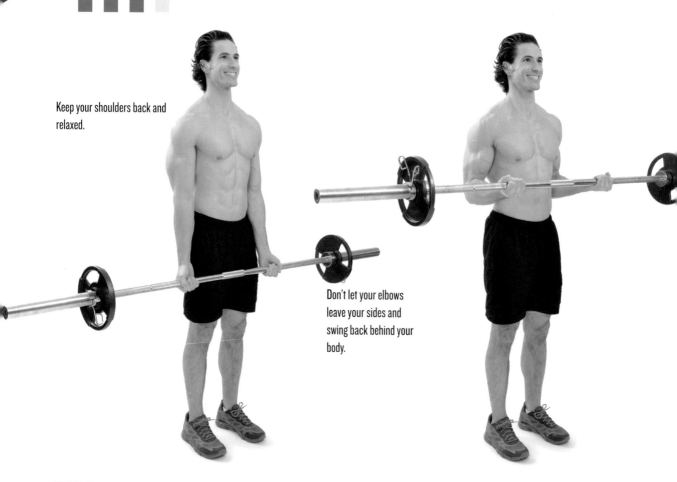

Keep your shoulders back and relaxed.

Don't let your elbows leave your sides and swing back behind your body.

 Stand with your feet shoulder width apart. Hold the barbell in front of your body with a supine (palms facing up) grip.

 Exhale as you bend at the elbows to curl the barbell up.

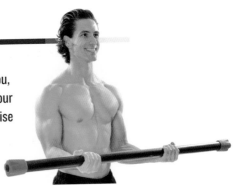

Remember, if the Olympic barbell is too heavy for you, you can always use a lighter fixed barbell. Also, if your wrists or elbows are strained, you can do this exercise with an EZ curl bar, which has grooves to give you more of a natural grip.

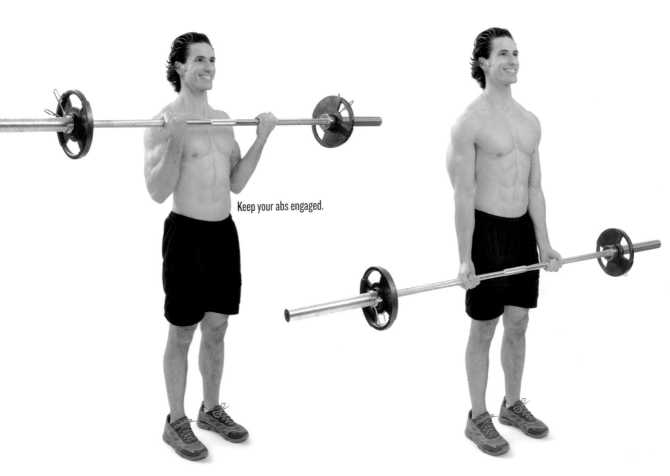

Keep your abs engaged.

 Squeeze your biceps when you're a little more than halfway up, and bring the barbell to the top of your chest.

4 Inhale as you control the barbell back to starting position.

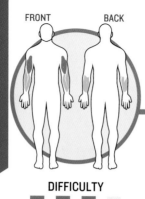

Barbell Bicep Reverse Curl

The barbell reverse curl not only challenges your hands and forearm muscles but also uses more of your core to control the weight of the barbell out in front of your body. This exercise strengthens your biceps and forearms.

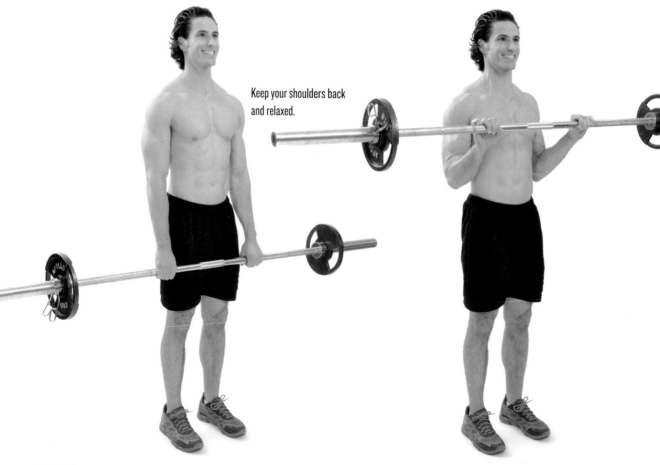

Keep your shoulders back and relaxed.

 Stand with your feet shoulder width apart. Using a prone grip (palms facing down), hold the barbell naturally in front of you.

 Exhale as you bend at the elbows to curl the barbell up.

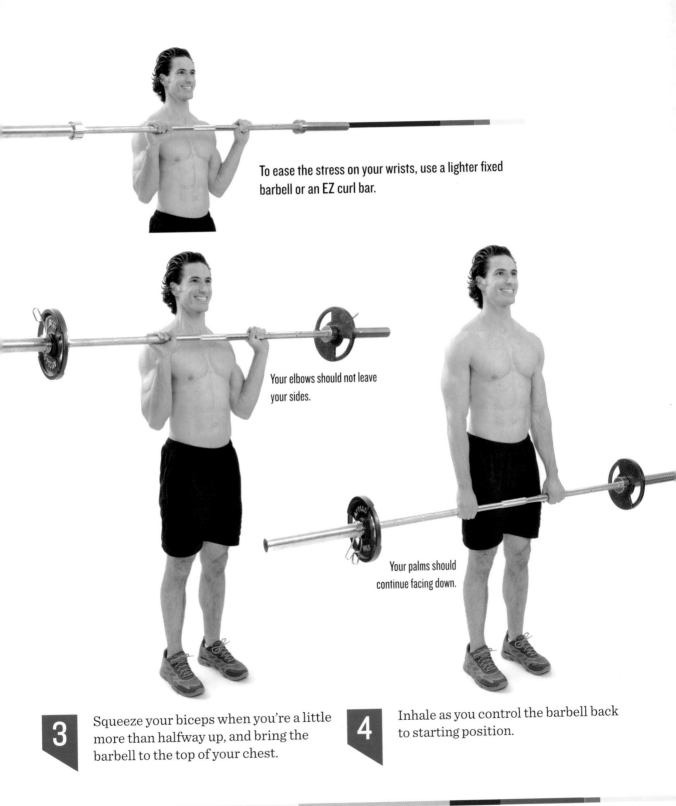

To ease the stress on your wrists, use a lighter fixed barbell or an EZ curl bar.

Your elbows should not leave your sides.

Your palms should continue facing down.

3 Squeeze your biceps when you're a little more than halfway up, and bring the barbell to the top of your chest.

4 Inhale as you control the barbell back to starting position.

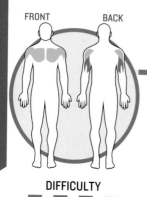

FRONT   BACK

Bench Dip

The bench dip is like a push-up for your arms. The addition of a bench allows you to use your legs help you complete the dip. This exercise targets your triceps while also giving your pecs and delts a nice stretch.

DIFFICULTY

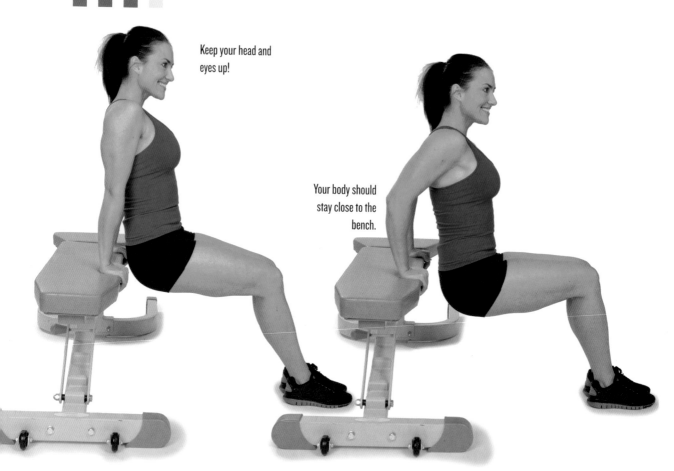

Keep your head and eyes up!

Your body should stay close to the bench.

 Place your hands behind you to hold you up, letting your hips hang off the bench. Your feet should be out in front of you on the floor.

 Inhale as you lower your body by bending at the elbows.

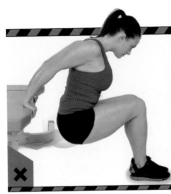

Be Careful!
Don't let your body get too far away from the bench. Otherwise, you'll put a dangerous strain on your shoulders and not work your triceps properly.

The height of the bench or step determines the difficulty of the exercise. The lower the bench, the less help you will have from your legs, and vice versa.

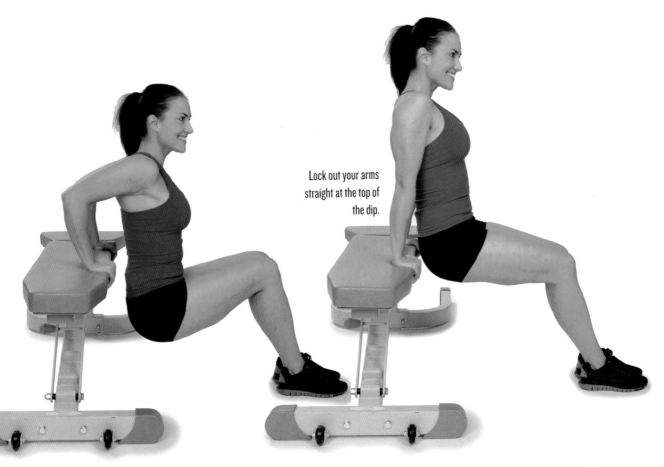

Lock out your arms straight at the top of the dip.

3 At the bottom of the dip, your elbows should be at a 90-degree angle.

4 Exhale as you push your body back up to starting position.

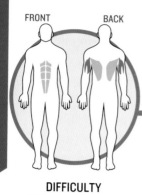

FRONT   BACK

DIFFICULTY

Barbell Tricep Skull Crusher

The barbell tricep skull crusher is a very advanced exercise that you must have the strength and technique to perform properly. This exercise targets your triceps, strengthens your upper body, and challenges the stabilizing muscles in your core.

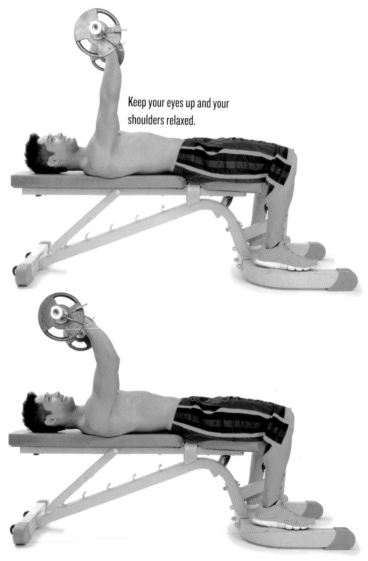

Keep your eyes up and your shoulders relaxed.

1 Lie on a bench with your arms straight up to hold the barbell. Your hands should be in a close, prone grip (palms facing forward).

2 Inhale as you bend your elbows to lower the barbell.

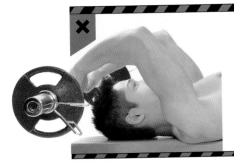

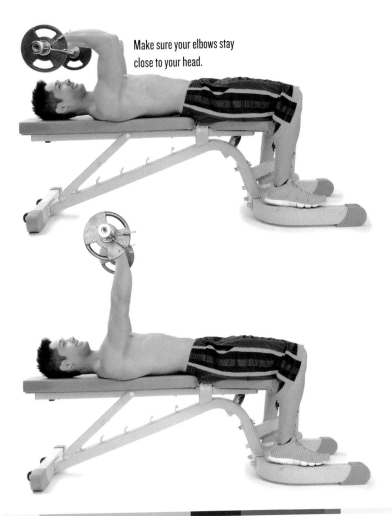

Make sure your elbows stay close to your head.

3 Create 90-degree angles with your elbows and engage your core.

4 Exhale as you extend your arms and press the barbell back up to starting position.

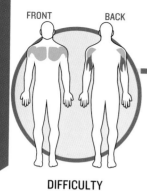

FRONT   BACK

Bodyweight Dip

The bodyweight dip is a progression of the bench dip and is second only to the pull-up as a great measurement of upper-body strength. It targets your triceps and provides a nice stretch for your delts and pecs.

DIFFICULTY

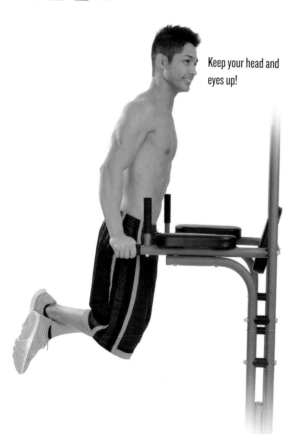

Keep your head and eyes up!

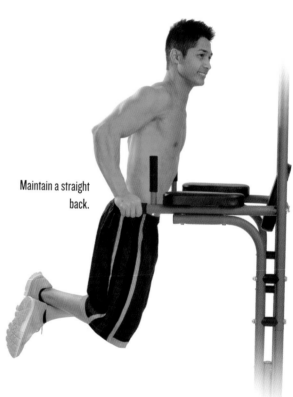

Maintain a straight back.

 Place your hands on the dip bars to hold yourself up, and allow your body to hang down naturally to the floor.

 Inhale as you lower your body by bending at the elbows.

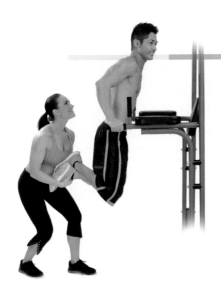

To get through those last few tough reps, have a buddy assist you by holding your feet. It could make all the difference in completing the exercise!

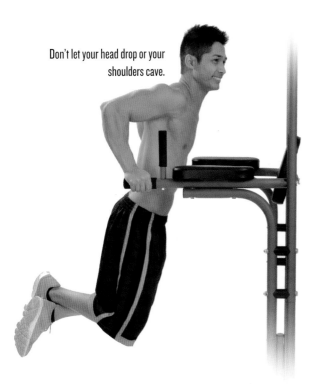

Don't let your head drop or your shoulders cave.

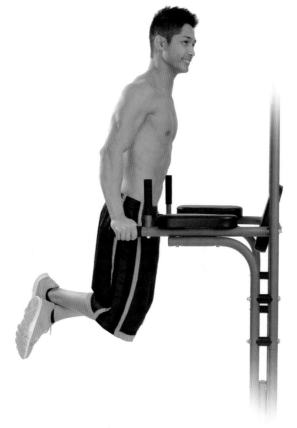

3 At the bottom of the dip, your elbows should be at a 90-degree angle.

4 Exhale as your push your body back up to starting position.

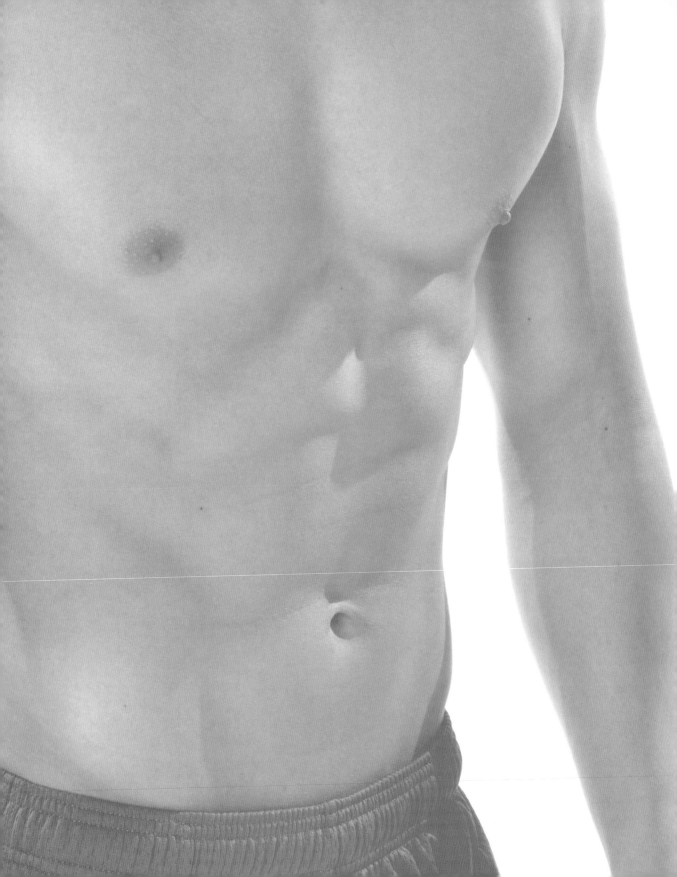

ABS

(Abdominals and Obliques)

Ah, the abs. You are always recruiting these amazing muscles. They help you sit up straight in your car as you drive and keep your body upright as you walk up or down a hill, making them extremely important muscles to condition and engage! Defined abs are also one of the most respected measures of a person's fitness level.

The **abdominals** are actually one very large muscle that's divided by connective tissue, giving it the "six-pack" look. The abdominals are responsible for all movements that include flexion in the spine, such as a crunch or sit-up. Your abdominals also help you with your breathing, especially exaggerated exhaling. The **obliques** are smaller muscles that run along the sides of your abdomen. These muscles are involved in external twisting and stretching. Most often, you use the abdominals and obliques simultaneously during core exercises and to stabilize while keeping your torso straight during both upper- and lower-body movements.

Having strong abs will help you become more efficient with the other exercises because you'll have a stronger base to begin with. You'll also find that doing simple, day-to-day routines—such as vacuuming the house, mowing the lawn, and playing with the kids in the yard—are easier with the help of conditioned abs.

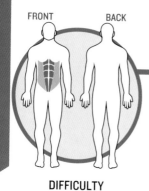

Basic Crunch

The basic crunch is a simple exercise that isolates the abdominals and obliques (torso). This version of the crunch requires you to only lift your shoulders off the floor, not sit up.

DIFFICULTY

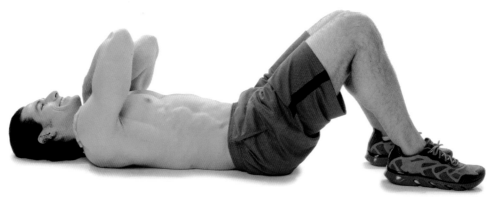

1 Lie on the floor with your back flat and your feet resting on the floor. Inhale as you stretch out your abs.

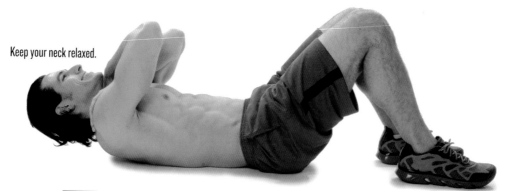

Keep your neck relaxed.

2 Exhale as your lift your shoulders off the floor to contract your abs.

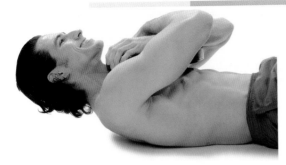

Variation
Challenge your core by holding a weight at chest level. This will force it to support the extra weight while you're doing the crunch.

Keep your eyes up.

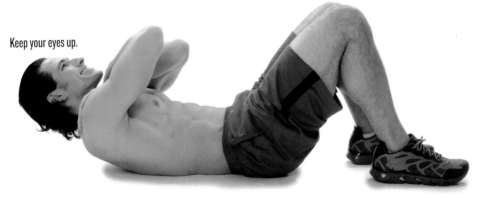

3 At the top of the crunch, when your shoulders are completely off the floor, squeeze your abs.

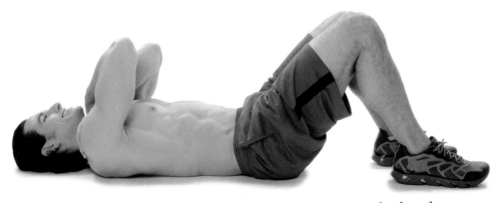

4 Inhale as you relax your shoulders and return back to the starting position.

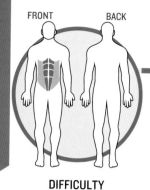

FRONT   BACK

ABS

DIFFICULTY

Stability Ball Crunch

Using a stability ball to do the crunch will add extra work to your recti abdominis and obliques (core) by challenging your balance. It also incorporates work from your erector spinae (lower back) to stabilize your position on top of the ball.

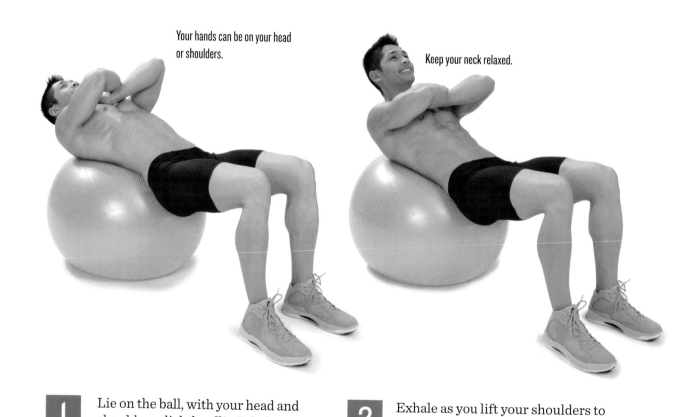

Your hands can be on your head or shoulders.

Keep your neck relaxed.

1 Lie on the ball, with your head and shoulders slightly off it. Inhale as you stretch out your abs.

2 Exhale as you lift your shoulders to contract your abs.

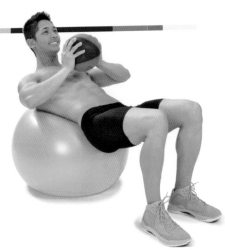

Variation

Like the basic crunch, you can hold a weight at chest level to add an extra challenge for your core.

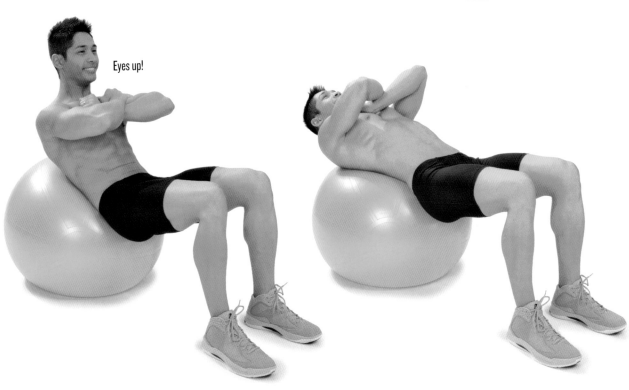

Eyes up!

 Squeeze your abs once you are at the top of the crunch. The ball should not move—only your upper body.

4 Inhale as you lower back to starting position.

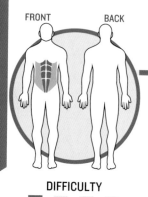

Bicycle Crunch

By crossing over your elbow to meet the opposite knee when doing this exercise, you create a circular, bike-peddling motion. The bicycle crunch involves constant movement from your arms and legs as you focus on contracting your abdominals (torso).

DIFFICULTY

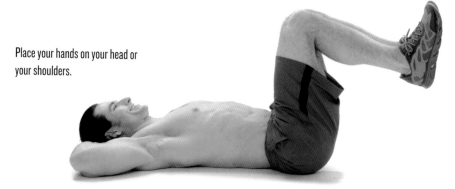

Place your hands on your head or your shoulders.

1 Lie on the floor with your knees bent and your feet off the ground to create a pelvic tilt. Inhale as you stretch out your abs.

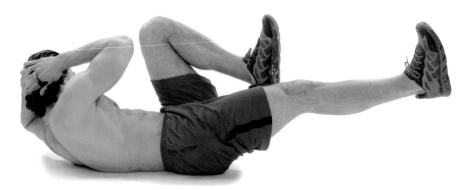

Keep your neck relaxed.

2 Exhale as you lift one shoulder and elbow and cross them over to meet the opposite knee.

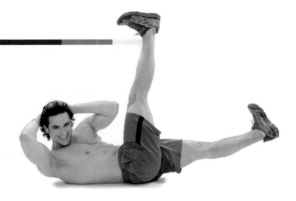

Variation

To progress this crunch, try it with straight legs! You can even do straight arms and reach for the opposite foot. Remember to keep your pelvis tilted in order to have proper form.

Eyes up!

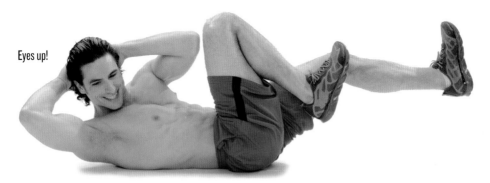

3 Repeat on the other side, keeping a constant crunch in your abs.

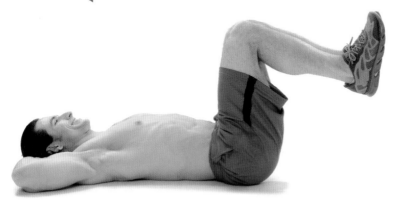

4 Relax as you rest your shoulders and return back to the floor.

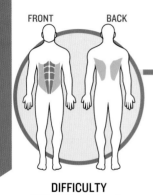

FRONT BACK

DIFFICULTY

Reverse Crunch

The reverse crunch is exactly what it sounds like: you work the same muscles as the regular crunch, but instead of lifting your shoulders off the floor or a bench, you lift your hips. It doesn't take much to feel the burn with this exercise! This exercise targets your abs.

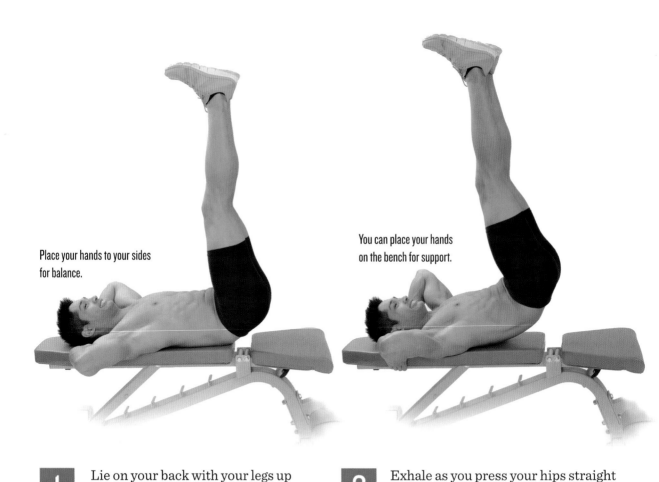

Place your hands to your sides for balance.

You can place your hands on the bench for support.

1 Lie on your back with your legs up while resting your head and shoulders on the bench. Inhale as you stretch out your abs.

2 Exhale as you press your hips straight up.

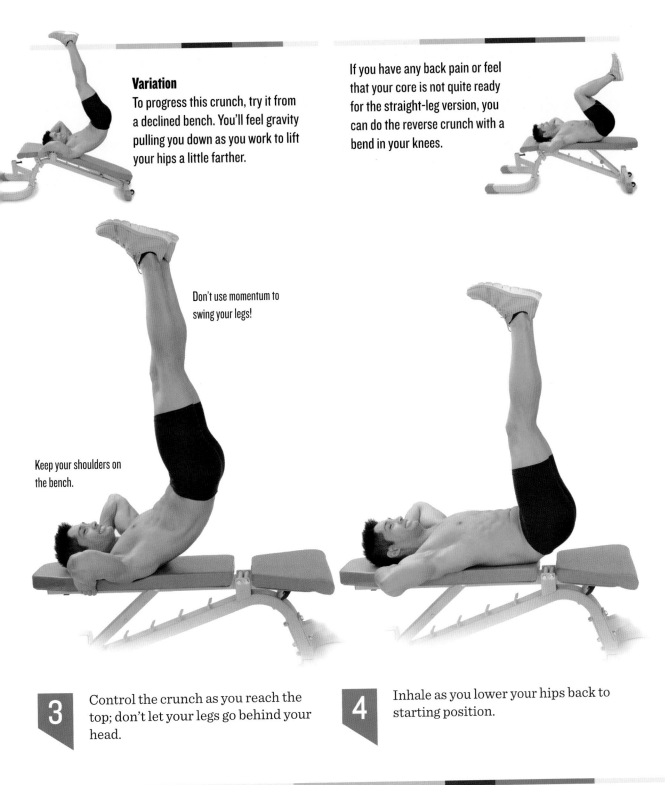

Variation
To progress this crunch, try it from a declined bench. You'll feel gravity pulling you down as you work to lift your hips a little farther.

If you have any back pain or feel that your core is not quite ready for the straight-leg version, you can do the reverse crunch with a bend in your knees.

Don't use momentum to swing your legs!

Keep your shoulders on the bench.

3 Control the crunch as you reach the top; don't let your legs go behind your head.

4 Inhale as you lower your hips back to starting position.

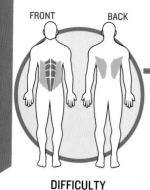

ABS

FRONT   BACK

DIFFICULTY

Cable Crunch Down

This crunch is probably very different from what you're used to—instead of lying on your back, you kneel and pull a weight down using a cable system. This move targets your abs along with the stabilizing muscles in your lower back.

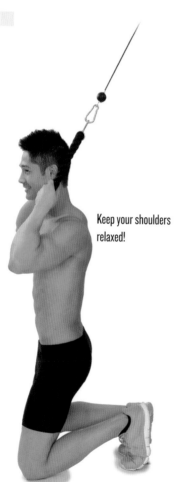

Keep your shoulders relaxed!

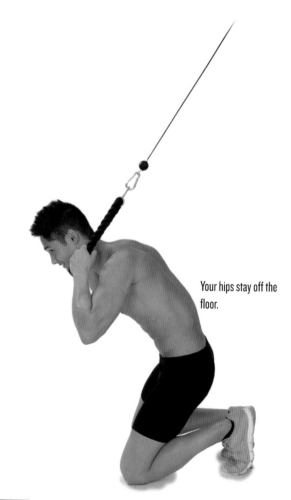

Your hips stay off the floor.

1 Kneel down, facing away from the cable system. Hold the cable handle at your shoulders, and inhale to stretch out your abs.

2 Exhale as you curl down toward your thighs, rounding your back as if you're doing a regular crunch.

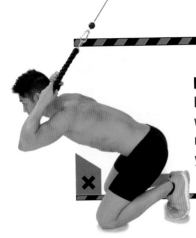

Be Careful!

If you feel like only your back muscles are being worked during this exercise, you are most likely not rounding down during the crunch. This can happen if you let your hips drop and keep your back straight.

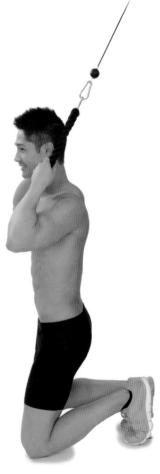

Your elbows should stay close to your thighs.

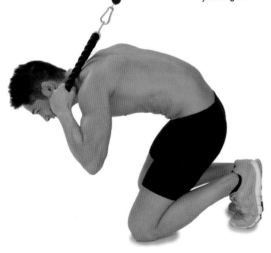

 3 At the bottom of the pull, squeeze your abs.

4 Inhale as you control the cable back to starting position.

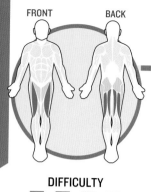

FRONT   BACK

Sit-Up

The sit-up is the big brother of the crunch. The beginning of this exercise mimics the crunch, but instead of a small movement, you sit all the way up. This exercise targets your abs.

DIFFICULTY

Your hands can be at your head or your shoulders.

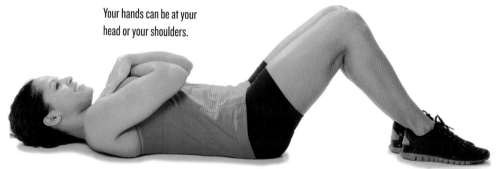

1 Lie on the floor with your back flat and your feet resting on the floor. Inhale as you stretch out your abs.

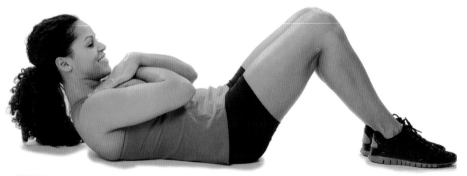

2 Exhale as your lift your shoulders off the floor to contract your abs.

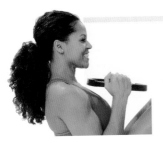

Variation
You can add an extra challenge for your core by holding a weight at chest level.

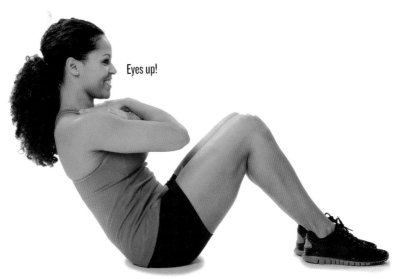

Eyes up!

3 Once you reach the fully upright seated position, squeeze your abs.

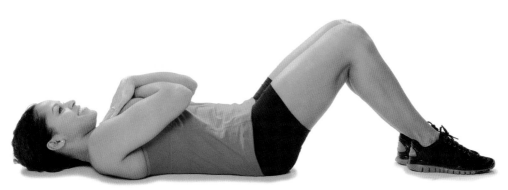

4 Inhale as you lower yourself back to the floor.

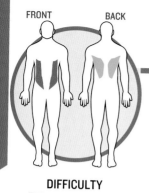

FRONT   BACK

Wood Chopper

In this fun yet challenging exercise, you move a weight through the air as if you are chopping wood. This incorporates rotation and flexibility in the torso, which gives your obliques a nice stretch.

DIFFICULTY

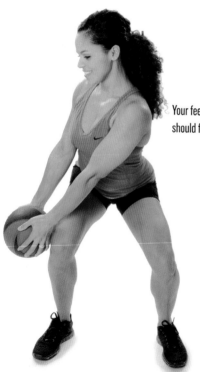

Your feet and shoulders should face forward.

Maintain straight arms.

 Hold a weight down at one side of your body. Stand with your feet shoulder width apart in a half squat.

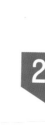 Inhale as you stretch your obliques by swinging the weight up to one side of your body.

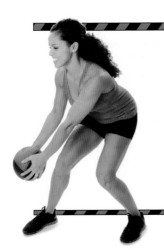

Be Careful!

This exercise can be dangerous to your knee and hip joints if you're not careful. Make sure you let your back foot pivot to allow your heel to come off the ground. Also, watch your knees as you chop down—don't let them move in or out.

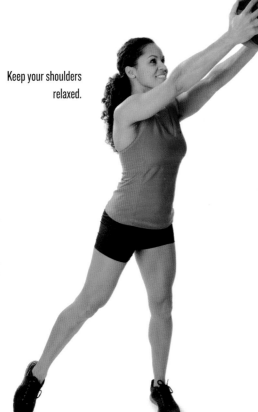

Keep your shoulders relaxed.

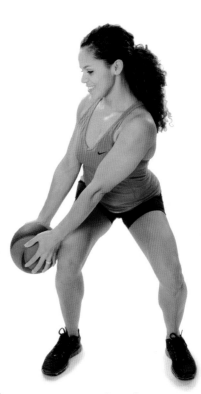

3 As your back heel comes off the floor, allow your torso to twist slightly to the side while your hips stay facing forward.

4 Exhale as you chop down toward the opposite knee to return back to starting position.

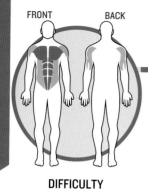

FRONT   BACK

DIFFICULTY

Mountain Climber

The mountain climber is a great exercise for many different muscles in your body. The push-up position strengthens all of your upper-body muscles—including your pecs, delts, traps, and lats—while the ability to hold yourself up challenges your abdominals.

1 Hold yourself up in a plank from your hands and feet. Inhale as you stretch and engage your abs.

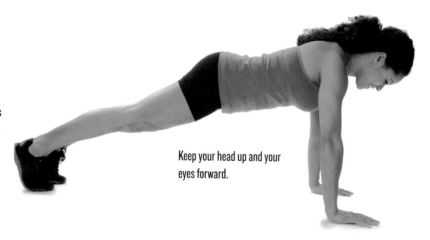

Keep your head up and your eyes forward.

Keep your arms straight! Don't let your shoulders drop.

2 Exhale as you bring one knee forward to the center of your body in a climbing position.

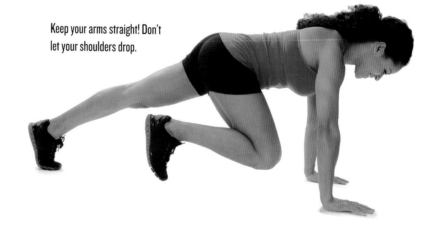

Don't let your hips drop.

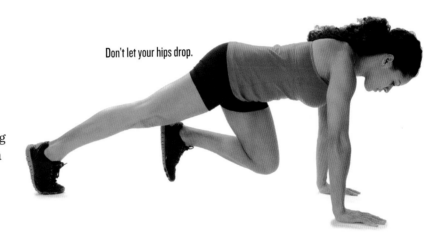

3 After your climbing foot reaches the other back in starting position, repeat with the opposite knee.

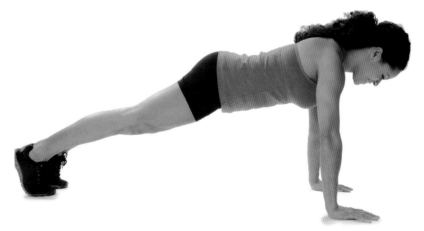

4 Inhale as you return your knee to starting position.

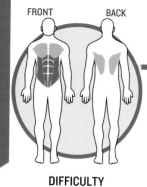

DIFFICULTY

Plank and Side Plank

The plank is a great core strengthener, while the side plank provides an extra stability challenge. I show two versions of the plank and the side plank—one from your hands and one from your elbow. These exercises target your core and require all of your upper body–stabilizing muscles.

Using your hands and feet, hold yourself up off the floor. Take deep breaths while contracting your abs to keep your body up in the plank.

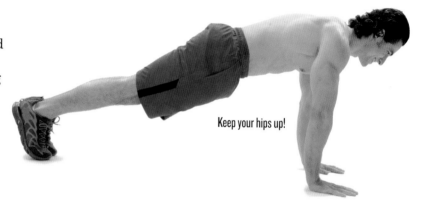

Keep your hips up!

Make sure your shoulders stay over your elbows.

Using your elbows and feet, hold yourself up off the floor. Take deep breaths while contracting your abs to keep your body up in the plank.

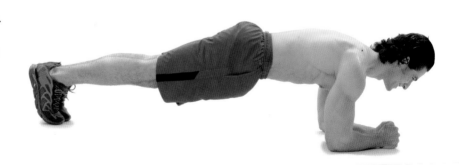

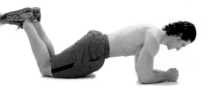

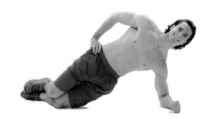

If you feel pressure in your lower back, you can drop your knees down to the floor and use them instead of your toes to support the plank or side plank. Even with this change, you should still feel your abs being worked.

Using your hand and feet, hold yourself up on one side of your body. Take deep breaths while contracting your abs to keep your body up in the plank.

Maintain straight legs.

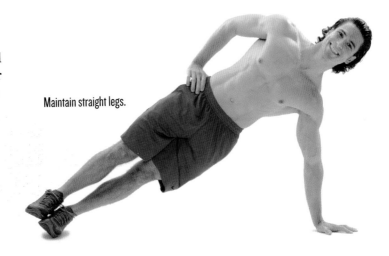

Using your elbow and feet, hold yourself up on one side of your body. Take deep breaths while contracting your abs to keep your body up in the plank.

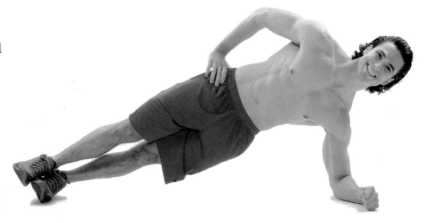

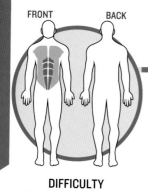

Stability Ball Pike

This exercise has many moving parts. You must stabilize your upper body while pulling in your legs with the help of your abs. This exercise targets your abs but is a great workout for your entire body.

DIFFICULTY

Your eyes should look slightly forward.

 With the stability ball at your feet, hold yourself in a push-up position. Inhale as you stretch and engage your core.

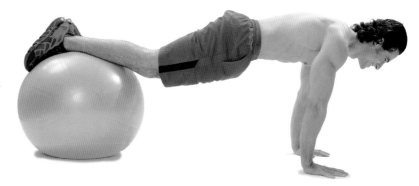

2 Exhale as you roll the ball toward the center of your body.

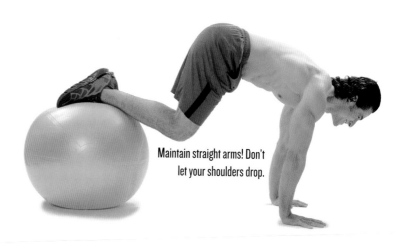

Maintain straight arms! Don't let your shoulders drop.

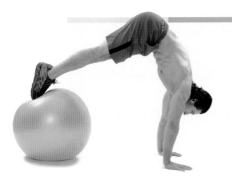

Variation
To progress this exercise, perform it with straight legs. Taking the bend out of your knees will require even more strength from your abs to roll the ball in.

Don't let your weight shift back onto the ball.

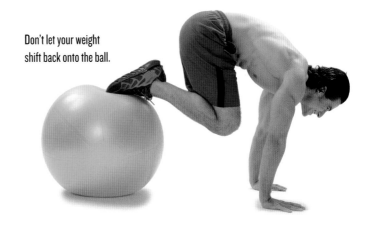

 3 When you reach the top of the roll, engage your abs to keep your hips up.

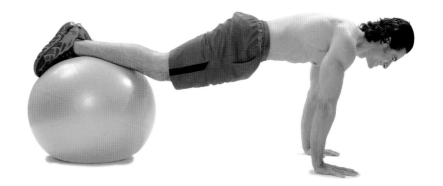

4 Inhale as you roll the ball back out to starting position.

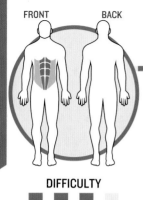

FRONT   BACK

V-Up

The V-up is like a sit-up without the lower-body stability. To do this move correctly, you pull your upper and lower body together using your core muscles for strength and balance. This exercise works your abs, obliques, and lower-back stabilizers.

DIFFICULTY

1 Lie on your back with your arms and legs stretched out. Inhale as you open up your abs.

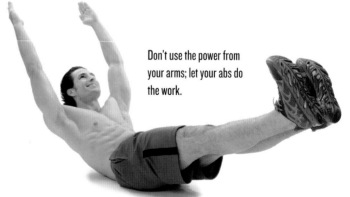

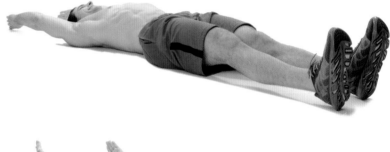

Don't use the power from your arms; let your abs do the work.

2 Exhale as you hinge at the hips to bring your shoulders toward your legs.

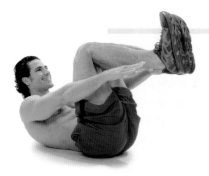

You can perform a similar move by simply crunching your shoulders and knees toward each other. The difference will be that your back will stay on the floor, providing you back support during the exercise.

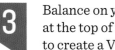

Keep your shoulders relaxed.

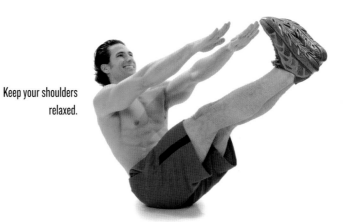

3 Balance on your hips at the top of the move to create a V with your body.

Let your back round down naturally.

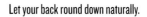

4 Inhale as you control your upper and lower body back down to starting position.

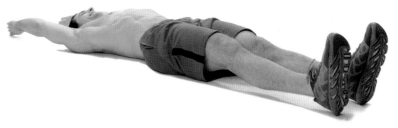

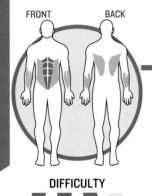

FRONT   BACK

Hanging Leg Lift

The hanging leg lift is a nice way to build strength in your midsection and hands. This exercise can be very tough if you can't hang from a pull-up position without assistance. It requires all your core muscles to control your legs while doing the lifts, along with help from your forearms and lats as you hang from the bar.

DIFFICULTY

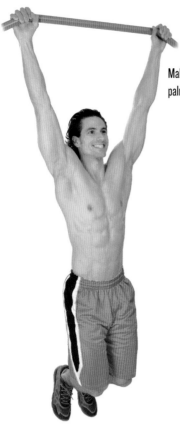

Make sure your palms face forward.

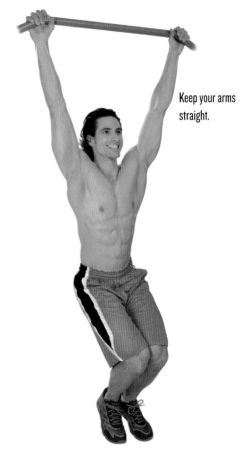

Keep your arms straight.

 1 With your arms stretched out and your legs naturally relaxed down, hold onto a pull-up bar. Inhale as you stretch your abs.

2 Exhale as you curl your knees up toward your chest to contract your abs.

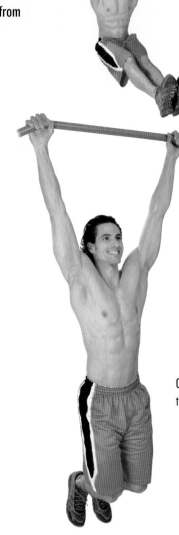

Variation

To give your core some extra work, do this move with straight legs. The farther away your feet are from your body, the harder they will be to lift!

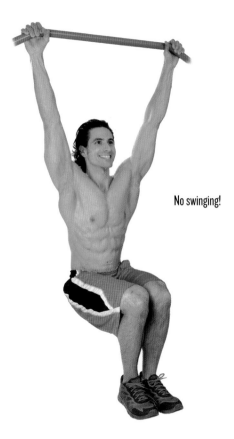

No swinging!

Control your legs on the way down.

 Squeeze your abs at the top of the crunch. Use control to avoid creating momentum.

 Inhale as you lower your legs back to starting position.

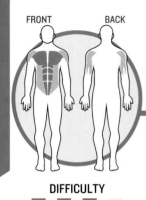

FRONT   BACK

DIFFICULTY

Stability Ball Mountain Climber

For an extra challenge to your core and upper body–stabilizing muscles, try doing the mountain climber with your hands on a stability ball. This exercise targets your pecs, delts, traps, lats, and abs.

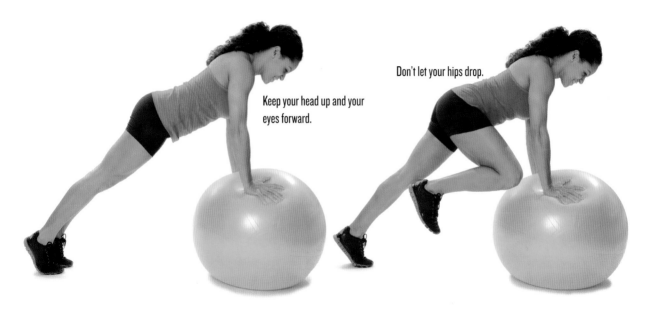

Keep your head up and your eyes forward.

Don't let your hips drop.

 With your hands on a stability ball and your feet on the floor, hold yourself up in a plank. Inhale as you stretch and engage your abs.

 Exhale as you bring one knee forward to the center of your body in a climbing position.

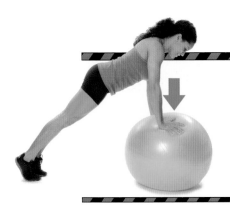

Be Careful!
Keep your bodyweight balanced over the top of the ball and not past it. If your weights shifts past the top, you could lose control and fall.

Keep your arms straight!
Don't let your shoulders drop.

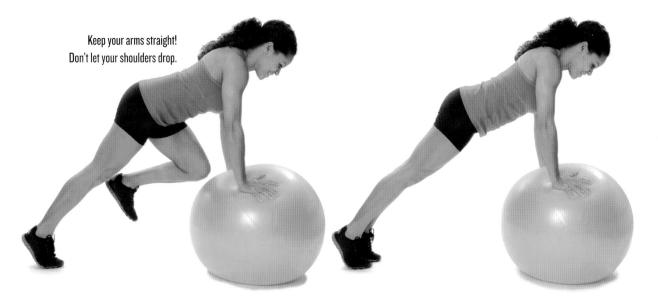

3 After your climbing foot reaches the other back in starting position, repeat with the opposite knee.

 4 Inhale as your return back to starting position.

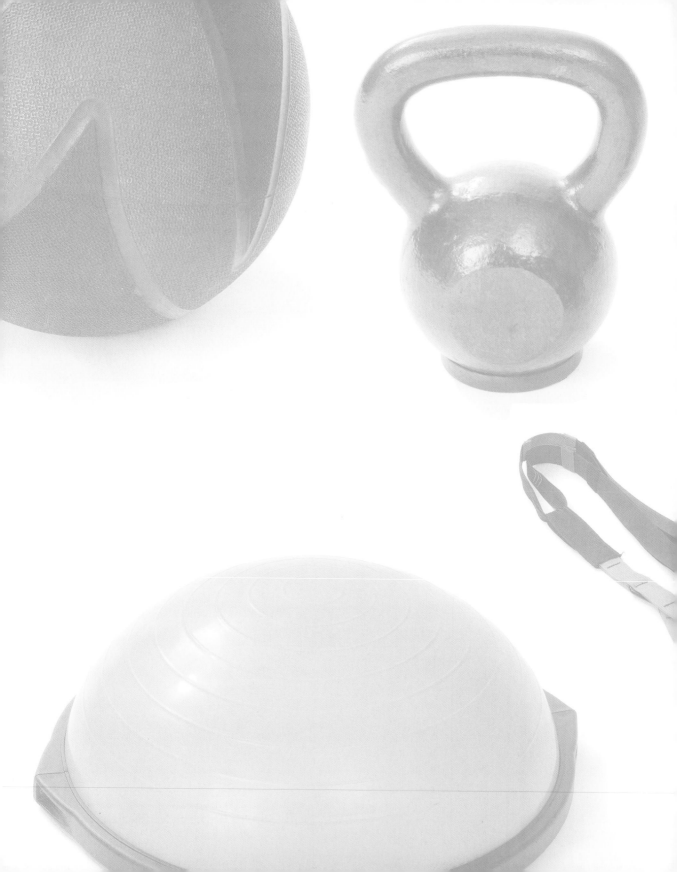

TRENDS

To add variety and complexity to your exercises, you can go beyond the standard weight-training equipment and check out some of the current trends. With the aid of a medicine ball, balance trainer, kettlebell, or suspension band system, you may find new and interesting ways to work different parts of your body.

A few words of caution, though: These exercises with special equipment don't take the place of the weight-training exercises featured earlier in the book. So before trying one of these trends, make sure you've learned the fundamentals of weight training and built up your core, upper-body, and lower-body strength. Also, in order to ensure proper form when trying these exercises, look into having a professional coach you. That way, you'll perform these exercises in a safe and effective manner.

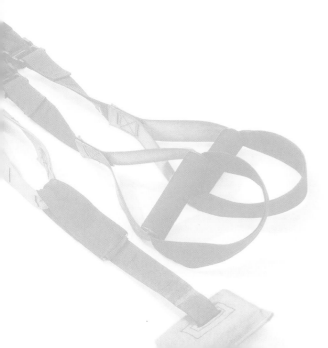

Medicine Balls

Medicine balls come in all different sizes and shapes, with variations in handles and difficulty of handling. They can be added into most weight-training exercises to either replace a free weight or simply make a bodyweight movement more challenging.

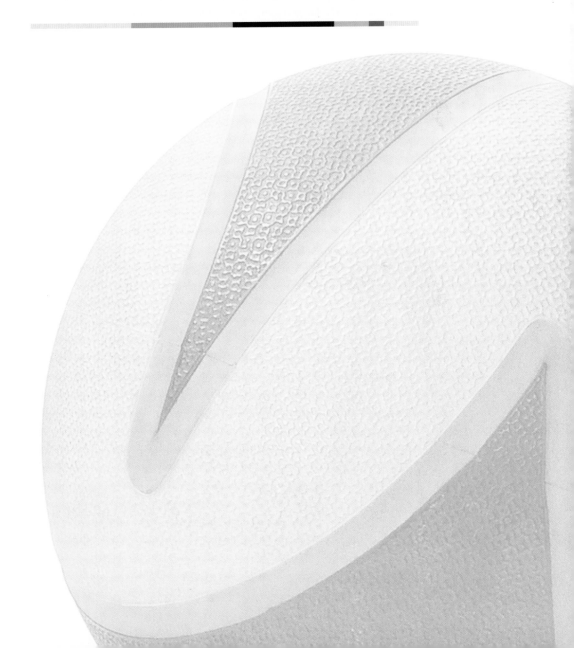

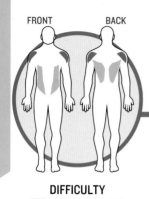

FRONT   BACK

DIFFICULTY

Medicine Ball Around the World

For around the world, you hold the medicine ball and bring it around your head in a continuous circular motion. This exercise targets the trapezius and deltoids (shoulders). You also get a little help from your pectorals (chest) and rhomboids (back).

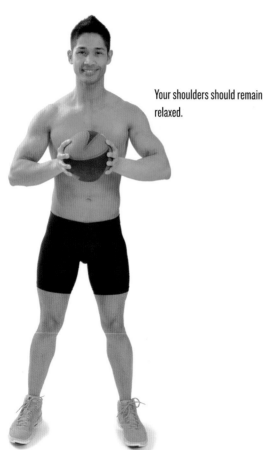

Your shoulders should remain relaxed.

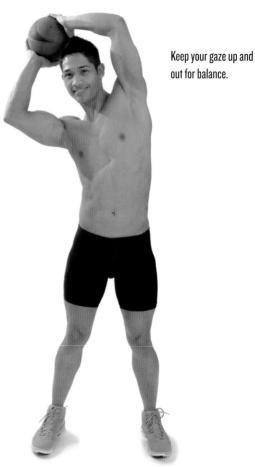

Keep your gaze up and out for balance.

1 With both hands, hold the medicine ball out in front of your chest.

2 Move the medicine ball to one side of your body, keeping it close to your head.

Make sure the movement in your torso is minimal so it doesn't become an abdominal exercise. The around the world move is more of a warm-up of the upper body that's great to incorporate at the beginning of an upper-body routine or in between sets.

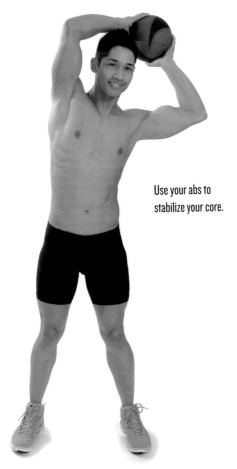

Use your abs to stabilize your core.

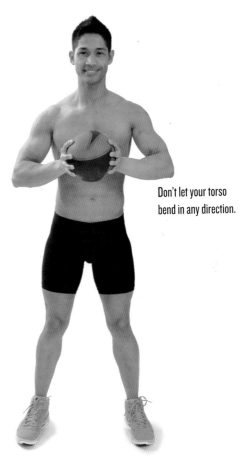

Don't let your torso bend in any direction.

3 Bring the medicine ball around your head using a continuous circular motion.

4 Once you have returned the medicine ball to the front, bring it back to starting position.

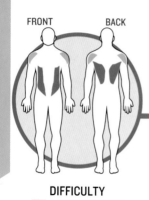

FRONT   BACK

DIFFICULTY

Medicine Ball Worship Stretch

The worship stretch is a very small stretch that requires focus and strength to do correctly. This version uses a medicine ball to lengthen and strengthen your abs and obliques (torso).

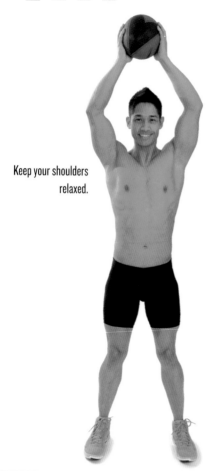

Keep your shoulders relaxed.

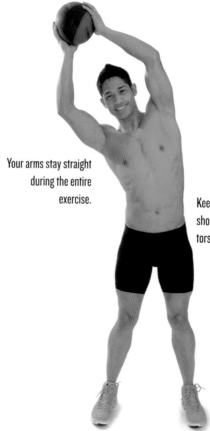

Your arms stay straight during the entire exercise.

Keep your hips still; you should only move your torso.

1 With both hands, hold the medicine ball straight above your head.

2 Inhale as you reach the medicine ball out and over to one side to stretch your obliques.

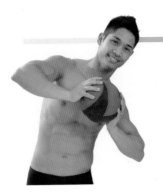

If your arms distract you from stretching your obliques, you can perform the worship stretch with your elbows bent and the medicine ball at your chest. This will allow you to focus more on the movement itself.

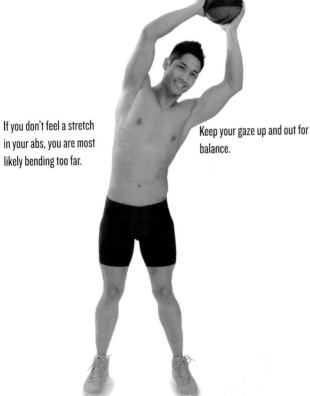

If you don't feel a stretch in your abs, you are most likely bending too far.

Keep your gaze up and out for balance.

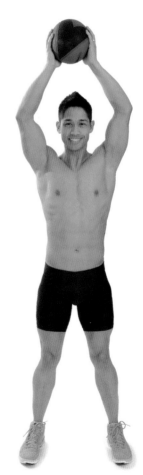

3 Exhale while passing through the center. Repeat the stretch to the other side, breathing deeply.

4 Bring the medicine ball back to starting position.

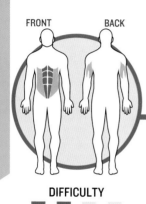

FRONT   BACK

DIFFICULTY

Medicine Ball Crunch Bounce

The crunch bounce not only strengthens your core but also incorporates torso rotation that will help with everyday tasks. Your core muscles in your abs and lower back stabilize you as you use power from your upper body to bounce the medicine ball on each side of your body.

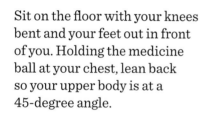

1 Sit on the floor with your knees bent and your feet out in front of you. Holding the medicine ball at your chest, lean back so your upper body is at a 45-degree angle.

Keep your neck relaxed and your shoulders down.

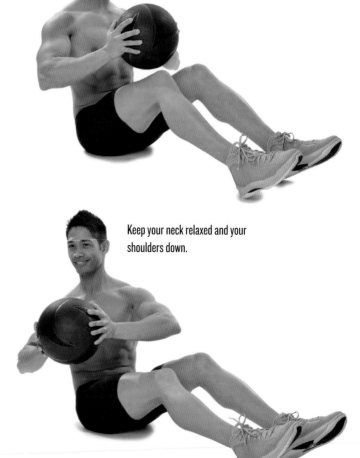

2 Exhale as you contract your abs and twist to one side.

If the bounce part of the exercise doesn't feel right to you, you can simply take it out and do the side-to-side movement without the bounce.

Your muscles will be worked the same way--you just won't have the pause on the side that the bounce gives you.

Allow your head and eyes to move naturally with your shoulders as you twist.

Stay in the leaned-back position for the entire exercise.

3 Bounce the medicine ball. Repeat the twist and bounce on the other side.

4 Return the medicine ball to starting position.

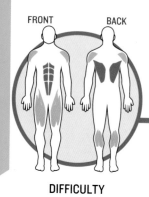

FRONT   BACK

DIFFICULTY

Medicine Ball Ball Slam

The ball slam is a powerful move for your abs. You hold the medicine ball with your hands, but use the power from your abs to perform the slam.

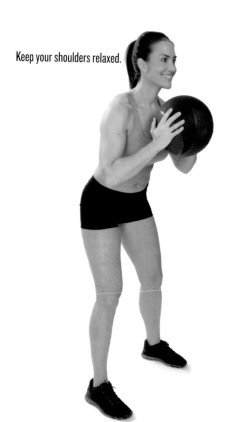

Keep your shoulders relaxed.

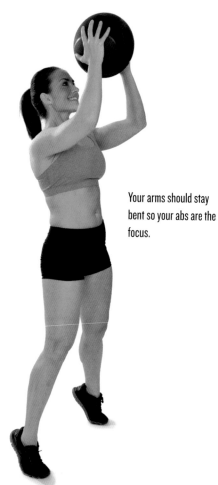

Your arms should stay bent so your abs are the focus.

Keep the medicine ball close to your body.

1 Stand with feet shoulder width apart. Hold the medicine ball at your chest.

2 Inhale as you stretch your abs by lifting the medicine ball just above eye level.

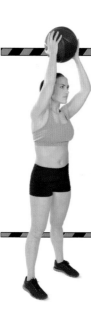

Be Careful!
Don't use your arms to perform this move. If your arms lift the medicine ball up and away from your body, you'll be using your arms and shoulders instead of your abs. By keeping the medicine ball close to your body, the power from your core will do all the work.

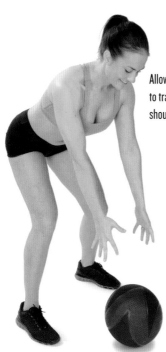

Allow your head and eyes to travel naturally with your shoulders.

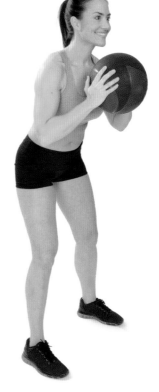

 Exhale as you contract your abs and bring your torso forward to slam the medicine ball down in front of you.

4 Catch the medicine ball on your way back to starting position.

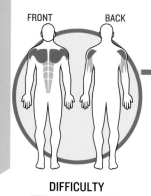

DIFFICULTY

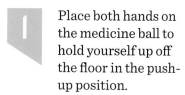

Medicine Ball Push-Up

Performing a push-up from a medicine ball—whether with one hand or both hands on it—adds a balance challenge that constantly uses the stabilizing muscles in your upper body. The two versions of this exercise also stretch your pecs differently than the standard version done on the floor. The medicine ball push-up targets your pecs, delts, triceps, and core muscles.

1 Place both hands on the medicine ball to hold yourself up off the floor in the push-up position.

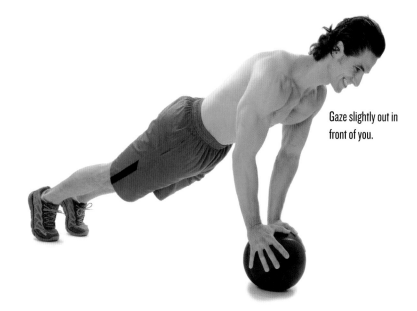

Gaze slightly out in front of you.

Keep your shoulders directly over the medicine ball.

2 Inhale as you descend into the push-up, creating a 90-degree angle with the elbows. Exhale as you ascend back to starting position.

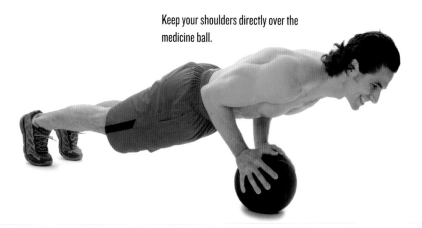

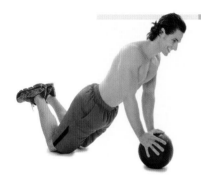

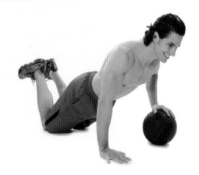

If you feel stress on your lower back or have trouble with your form, you can drop your knees down to the floor to perform a kneeling push-up.

1 Place one hand on the medicine ball and the other hand flat on the floor to hold yourself up in the push-up position.

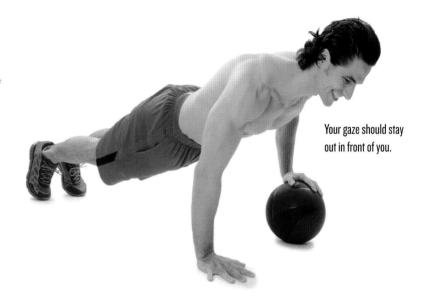

Your gaze should stay out in front of you.

Keep your shoulders over your hands.

2 Inhale as you descend into the push-up, creating a 90-degree angle in the elbows. Exhale as you ascend back to starting position.

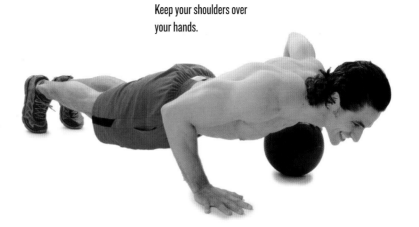

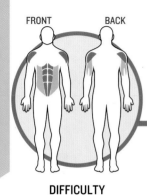

FRONT   BACK

DIFFICULTY

Medicine Ball Sit-Up Press

The addition of a medicine ball at chest level for the sit-up press provides a great workout for your abs because of the extra weight. This exercise also incorporates your pecs and delts by adding a press at the top of the movement.

1 Lie on the floor with your knees bent and your feet resting on the floor. Hold the medicine ball at your chest, and inhale as you stretch your abs.

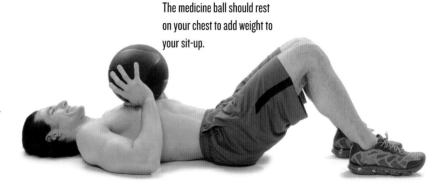

The medicine ball should rest on your chest to add weight to your sit-up.

2 Exhale as your lift your shoulders off the floor to contract your abs.

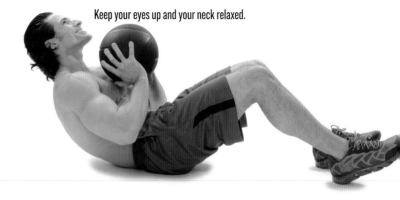

Keep your eyes up and your neck relaxed.

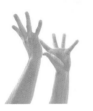

Variation
Add some power to this exercise by tossing the medicine ball at the top instead of pressing it. The explosive toss will give your upper body an extra challenge.

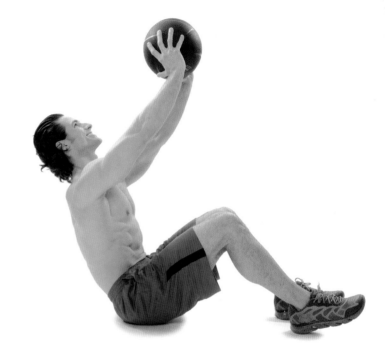

3 Once you are at the top of the sit-up, press the medicine ball up.

4 Inhale as you lower yourself back to starting position.

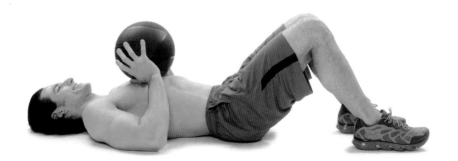

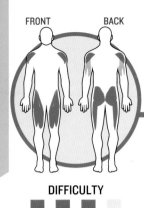

Medicine Ball Sun God Squat

Similar to the sumo squat, the sun god squat requires a wide stance and targets your glutes, hamstrings, and quads. With the addition of a medicine ball press, you also incorporate your upper body, including your delts, traps, and triceps.

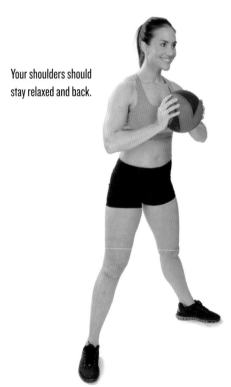

Your shoulders should stay relaxed and back.

Engage your abs to keep your back straight.

Maintain your weight in your heels.

1 Stand with your feet outside of your shoulders for a strong, wide stance. Hold the medicine ball with both hands at your chest.

2 Inhale as you descend into the squat, creating a 90-degree angle with your knees.

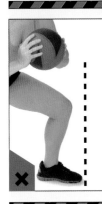

Be Careful!

Always be aware of the angles in your joints to protect them from injury. For squats, you should take care not to let your knees go past your toes.

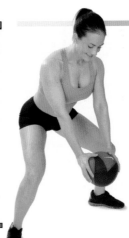

Variation

Bounce the medicine ball down to the center of your body when you are in the squat. This keeps your body in the squat position for a moment longer and adds power from your upper body and core to bounce the medicine ball.

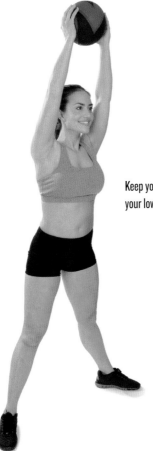

Keep your eyes up to protect your lower back from arching.

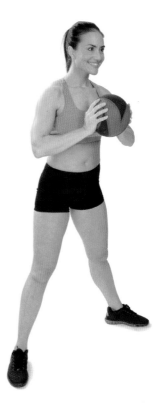

3 Exhale as you ascend back to standing position and press the medicine ball straight up.

4 Inhale as you bring the medicine ball back to starting position.

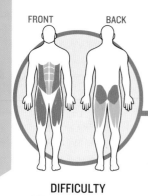

FRONT BACK

DIFFICULTY

Medicine Ball Lunge and Twist

The lunge and twist requires great focus and balance as you try to stay stable while twisting with the medicine ball. This exercise targets your quads, glutes, and hamstrings. You also give your core extra work with the weighted twist.

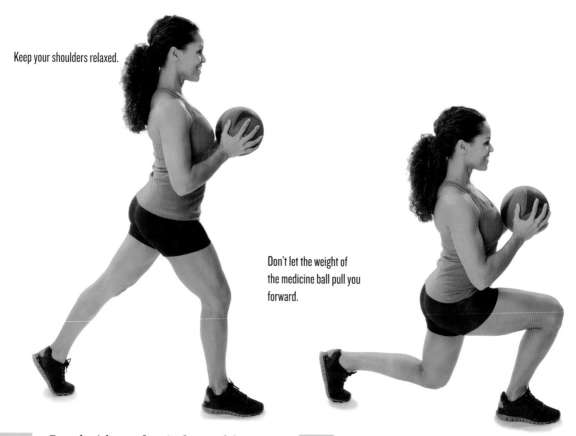

Keep your shoulders relaxed.

Don't let the weight of the medicine ball pull you forward.

1 Stand with one foot in front of the other, with equal balance between them, and bring your back heel off the ground. Hold the medicine ball with both hands at your chest.

2 Inhale as you lower into the lunge, creating a 90-degree angle with your knees.

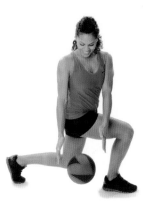

Variation

After twisting to the side, try bouncing the medicine ball. This will keep you down in the lunge position for a moment longer while your upper body uses power to bounce the medicine ball.

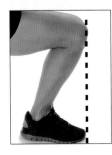

Be Careful!

Don't let your knee extend past your toes during the lunge. Your knee joint won't be able to support the weight of your body, which could result in injury.

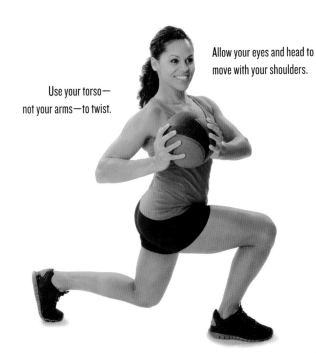

Use your torso—not your arms—to twist.

Allow your eyes and head to move with your shoulders.

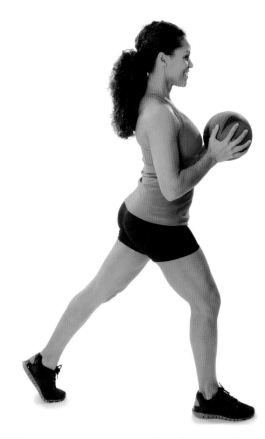

3 Exhale as you contract your abs and twist toward the leg out in front.

4 Inhale as you ascend back to starting position.

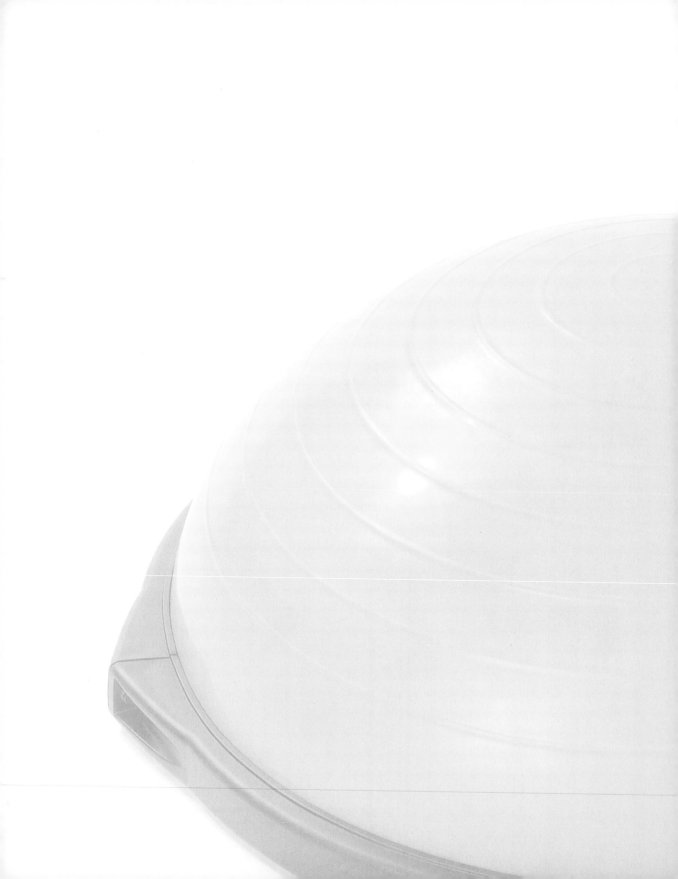

Balance Trainers

Add a stability challenge to your basic exercises by using the round or flat side of a balance trainer. Because you have to engage the stabilizing muscles in your lower body, upper body, and core for control on top of this piece of equipment while also completing the exercise, you'll burn more calories.

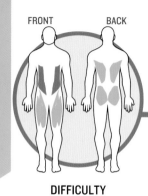

FRONT   BACK

DIFFICULTY

Balance Trainer Wood Chopper

Doing the wood chopper on a balance trainer requires more focus on balance and full-body awareness because you're constantly trying to stay stable. This exercise improves the stabilizing muscles in your lower body and core, rotation and flexibility in your torso, and strength in your obliques.

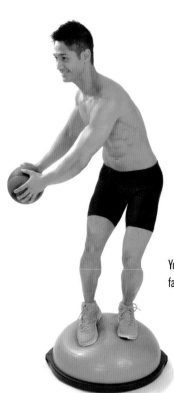

Keep your arms straight.

Your feet and shoulders should face forward.

 Hold a medicine ball (or your weight of choice) down at one side of your body. Stand comfortably on the round side of the balance trainer in a half squat.

 Inhale as you stretch your obliques by swinging the weight up to one side of your body.

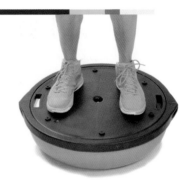

Variation

For an even greater stability challenge, flip the balance trainer over to perform the wood chopper from the flat side.

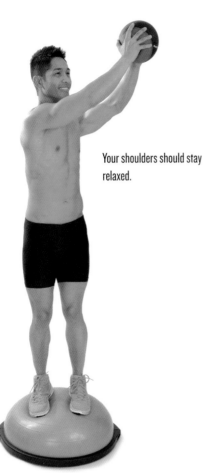

Your shoulders should stay relaxed.

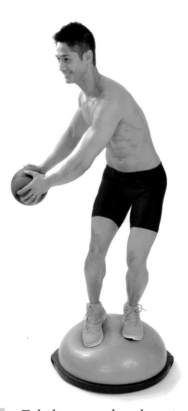

3 Allow your torso to twist slightly to the side, keeping your hips facing forward.

4 Exhale as you chop down toward the opposite knee to return back to starting position.

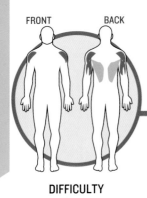

FRONT   BACK

DIFFICULTY

Balance Trainer Crab Walk

In the crab walk, you use your arms to walk around the balance trainer, similar to the movement of a crab. This exercise challenges the stabilizers in your upper body and tests the strength of your triceps and delts.

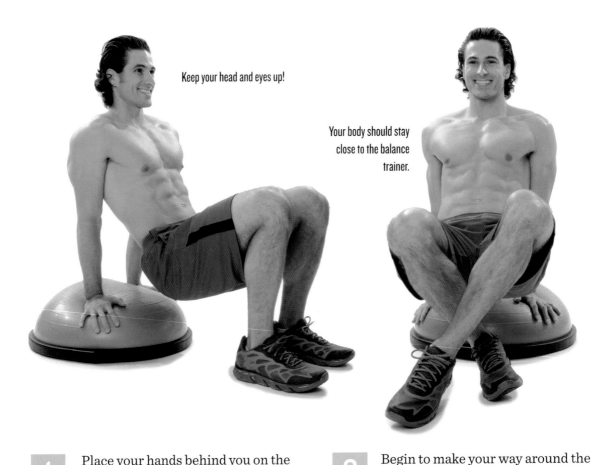

Keep your head and eyes up!

Your body should stay close to the balance trainer.

1 Place your hands behind you on the balance trainer, keeping your hips up off the floor. Place your feet out in front of you on the floor.

2 Begin to make your way around the balance trainer, with your hands moving along the balance trainer while your feet walk on the floor.

Be Careful!
Make sure you keep your body close to the balance trainer as you move around it. Getting too far away from the balance trainer can cause unwanted strain on your shoulders and stress your elbow joints.

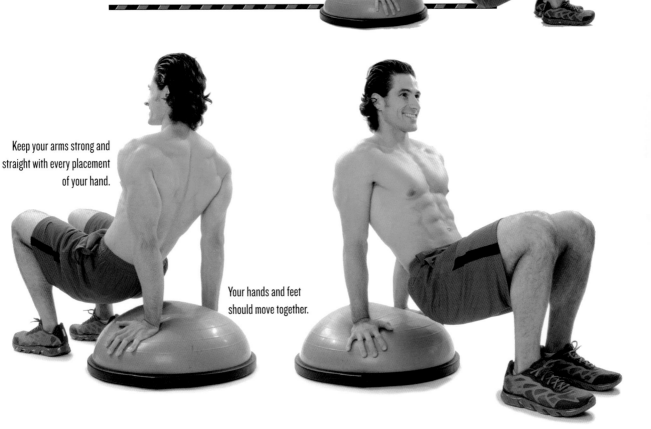

Keep your arms strong and straight with every placement of your hand.

Your hands and feet should move together.

3 Make your way around the balance trainer in a circular motion.

4 Complete the circle around the balance trainer and return to starting position.

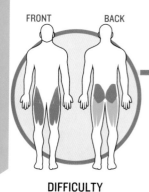

FRONT   BACK

DIFFICULTY

Balance Trainer Squat

Doing squats on a balance trainer—whether on the round side or the flat side—adds a challenge to your core and the stabilizing muscles in your legs because you have to perform the exercise as you try to keep your balance on the instable ball. This exercise targets the major muscles of your lower body, including your glutes, hamstrings, and quads.

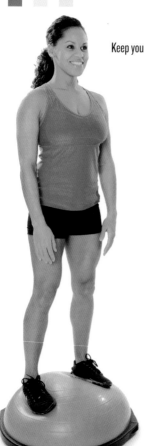

Keep your eyes up for balance!

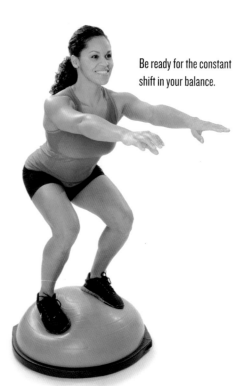

Be ready for the constant shift in your balance.

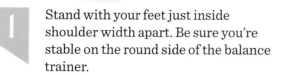

1 Stand with your feet just inside shoulder width apart. Be sure you're stable on the round side of the balance trainer.

2 Inhale as you descend into the squat, creating a 90-degree angle with your knees. Exhale as you ascend back to starting position.

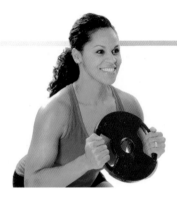

Variation
For an even greater challenge to your core, hold a weight at your chest.

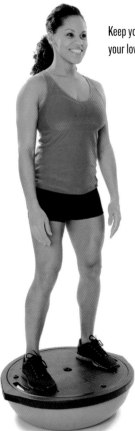

Keep your eyes up to protect your lower back from arching.

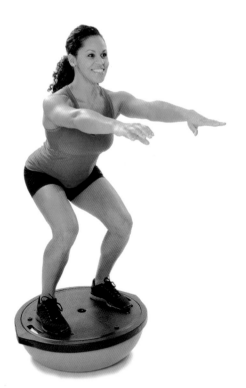

1 Stand with your feet just inside shoulder width apart. Be sure you're stable on the flat side of the balance trainer.

2 Inhale as you descend into the squat, creating a 90-degree angle with your knees. Exhale as you ascend back to starting position.

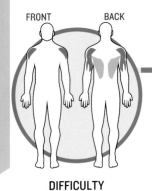

DIFFICULTY

Balance Trainer Dip

Doing the dip from a balance trainer is a much smaller movement than the bodyweight dip or even the bench dip because you're closer to the ground. While you balance on the round side of the balance trainer, you recruit extra work from the stabilizers in your upper body along with strength from your triceps and delts.

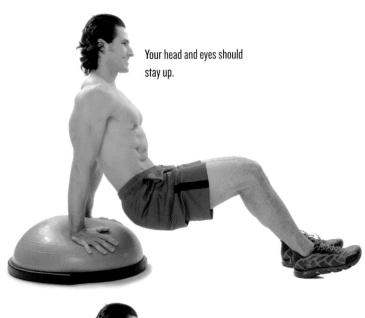

Your head and eyes should stay up.

1 Place your hands behind you on the balance trainer, keeping your hips up off the floor. Place your feet out in front of you on the floor.

2 Inhale as you lower your body by bending at the elbows.

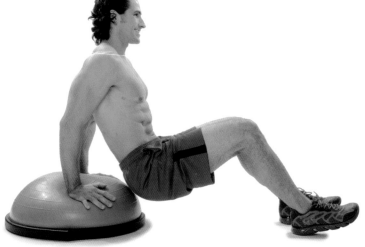

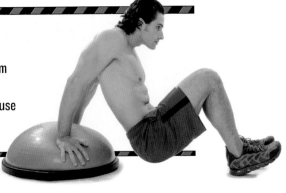

Be Careful!
Don't let yourself get too far away from the balance trainer. Otherwise, you could stress your elbow joints and cause unwanted strain on your shoulders.

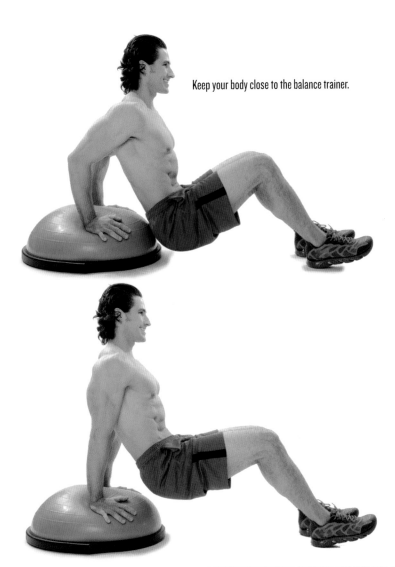

Keep your body close to the balance trainer.

3 At the bottom of the dip, your elbows should be at a 90-degree angle.

4 Exhale as your push your body back up to starting position.

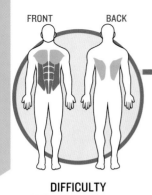

FRONT   BACK

DIFFICULTY

Balance Trainer Plank

Performing the plank from a balance trainer adds an extra challenge to the stabilizing muscles in your upper body and core, including your chest, shoulders, arms, and abs. The abdominals and obliques are constantly challenged during all of these versions of the plank.

Hold yourself up off the balance trainer by placing your elbows on the round side and your toes on the ground.

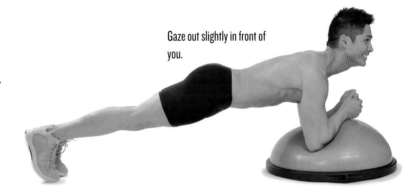

Gaze out slightly in front of you.

For a modified version that takes some pressure off your lower back, hold yourself up off the balance trainer by placing your elbows on the round side and your knees on the ground.

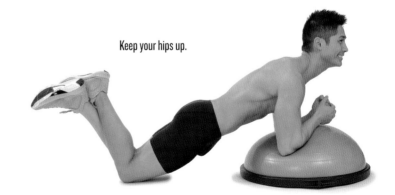

Keep your hips up.

Hold yourself up off the balance trainer by placing your elbows on the flat side of the balance trainer and your toes on the ground.

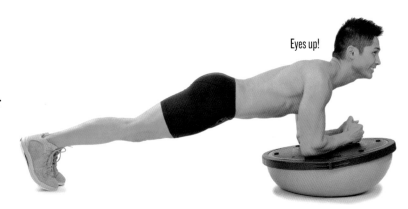

Eyes up!

For a modified version that takes some pressure off your lower back, hold yourself up off the balance trainer by placing your elbows on the flat side and your knees on the ground.

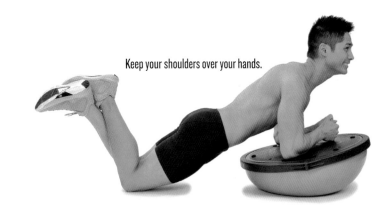

Keep your shoulders over your hands.

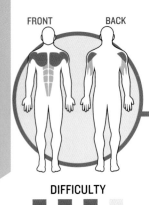

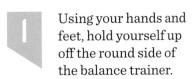

Balance Trainer Push-Up

Performing a push-up on the round side or flat side of a balance trainer adds an extra challenge to the stabilizing muscles in your upper body and core, including your pecs, delts, triceps, and abs.

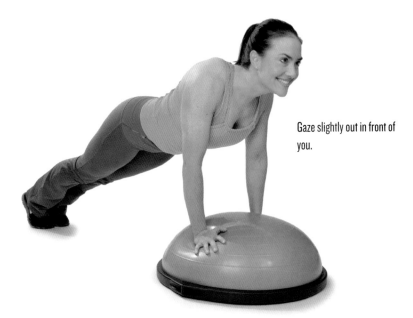

Gaze slightly out in front of you.

1 Using your hands and feet, hold yourself up off the round side of the balance trainer.

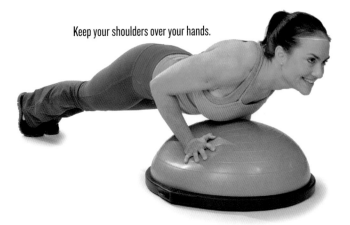

Keep your shoulders over your hands.

2 Inhale as you descend into the push-up, creating a 90-degree angle with your elbows. Exhale as you ascend back to starting position.

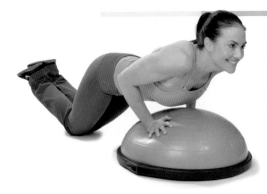

Drop your knees down to the floor to perform a kneeling push-up on the balance trainer if your lower back is too stressed or if you're having trouble with your form doing a regular push-up.

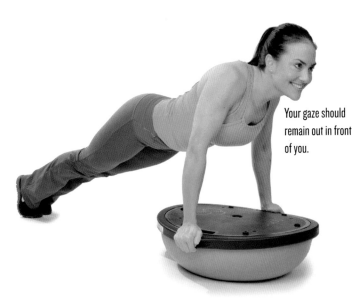

Your gaze should remain out in front of you.

1 Using your hands and feet, hold yourself up off the flat side of the balance trainer.

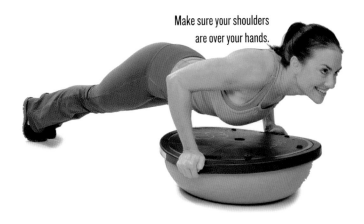

Make sure your shoulders are over your hands.

2 Inhale as you descend into the push-up, creating a 90-degree angle with your elbows. Exhale as you ascend back to starting position.

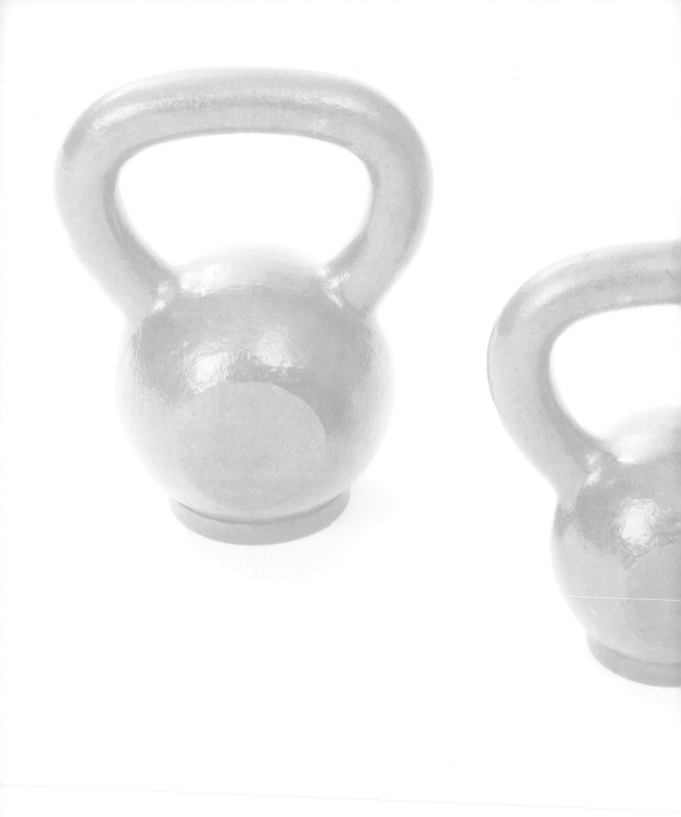

Kettlebells

Kettlebells uniquely bring together anaerobic and aerobic exercise because they both help you build muscle and condition your cardiovascular strength. These cannonball-like pieces of equipment use multiple muscles and joints during any single exercise, so you get a very complex and challenging workout.

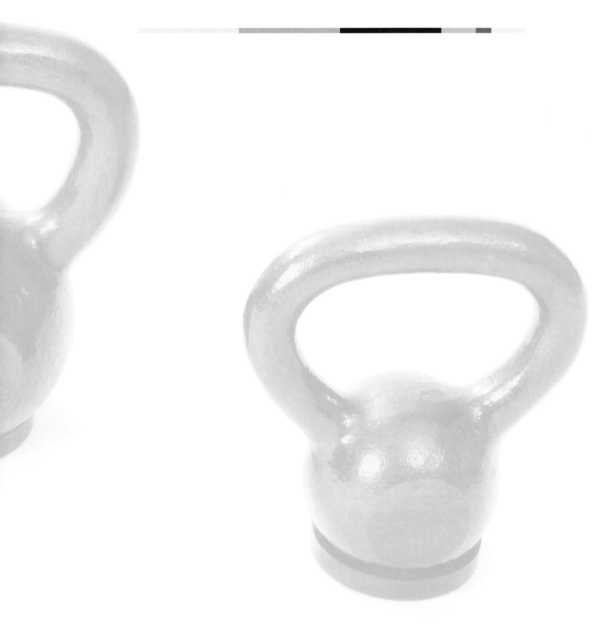

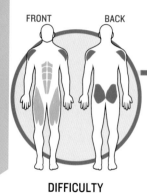

Kettlebell Figure 8

In the figure 8, you pass the kettlebell through your legs using core stability while holding a deep athletic stance. This is a fluid-moving exercise that requires upper- and lower-body awareness. This exercise targets your abdominals and spine erectors (core) and your deltoids and trapezius muscles (shoulder girdle).

DIFFICULTY

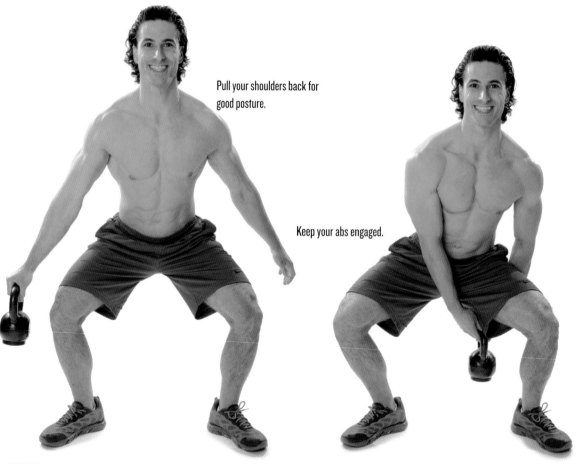

Pull your shoulders back for good posture.

Keep your abs engaged.

1 Stand in a deep athletic stance, with your feet just beyond shoulder width apart. Hold a kettlebell in one hand.

2 Bring the kettlebell across your body to pass under your leg to your other hand.

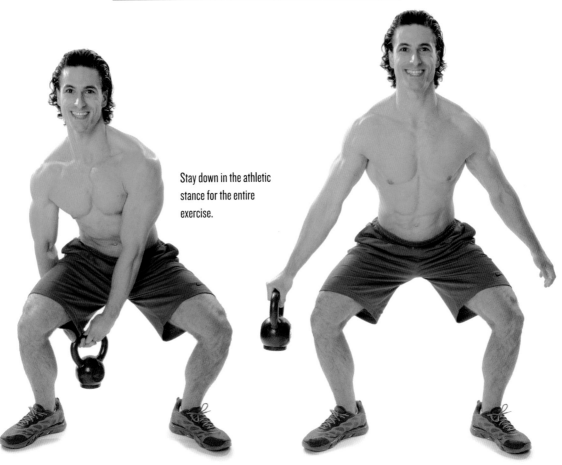

Stay down in the athletic stance for the entire exercise.

3 Repeat from the other side, breathing deeply.

4 The kettlebell should now be back at starting position.

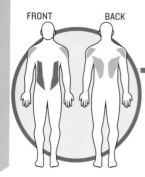

Kettlebell Windmill

The windmill is like a combination of a stretch and a side crunch done standing up. This exercise targets your obliques (sides of your torso).

DIFFICULTY

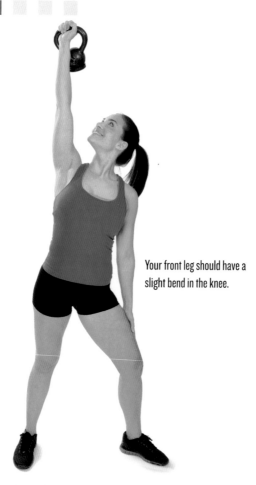

Your front leg should have a slight bend in the knee.

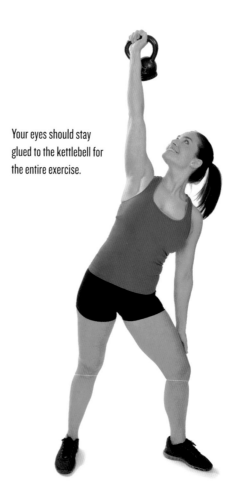

Your eyes should stay glued to the kettlebell for the entire exercise.

1 Stand with your feet just beyond shoulder width apart. Hold a kettlebell in one hand, and stretch your arm straight up to the ceiling.

2 Inhale as your hand slides down your front leg to stretch your obliques.

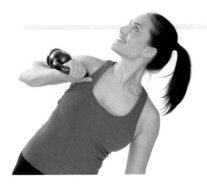

If you find it hard to keep your arm straight during the windmill, you can do this exercise with a bent elbow and the kettlebell at your shoulder. The form is the same for the rest of your body and allows you to still focus on stretching your obliques.

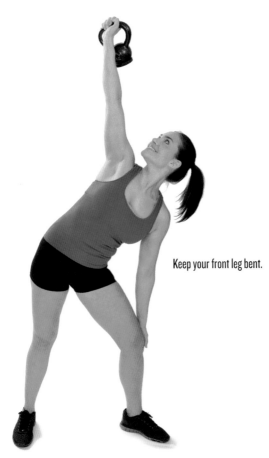

Keep your front leg bent.

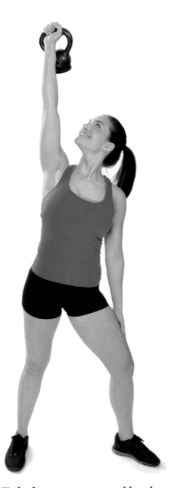

3 As your torso bends to the side, keep the arm holding the kettlebell directly vertical.

4 Exhale as you ascend back to starting position.

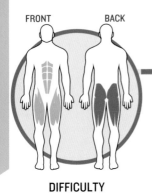

FRONT   BACK

DIFFICULTY

Kettlebell Swing

The swing is fundamental in kettlebell training. You use power and momentum from your hips and core to swing the kettlebell up into the air. Your glutes do most of the work, while your abs control the kettlebell midmove to allow it to fall back to the ground.

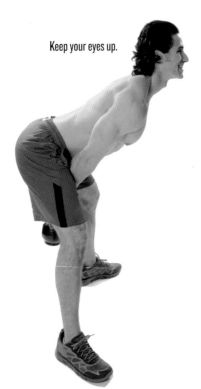

Keep your eyes up.

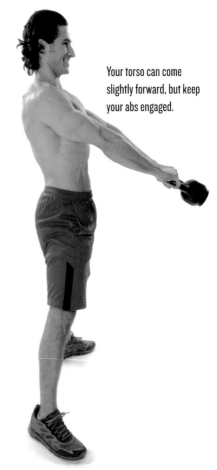

Your torso can come slightly forward, but keep your abs engaged.

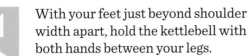

1 With your feet just beyond shoulder width apart, hold the kettlebell with both hands between your legs.

2 Using the power from your legs, explode the kettlebell up into the air by extending your hips forward like you would during a deadlift.

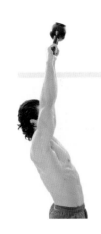

You can also do the kettlebell swing up past eye level or even over your head in a full swing. Take care to control the swing, and know when to stop it to let the downward motion begin.

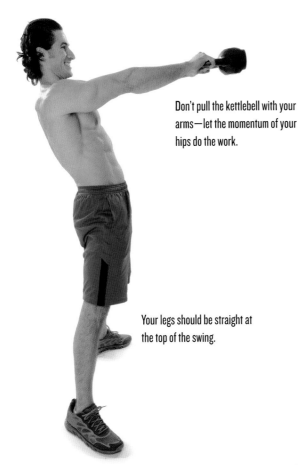

Don't pull the kettlebell with your arms—let the momentum of your hips do the work.

Your legs should be straight at the top of the swing.

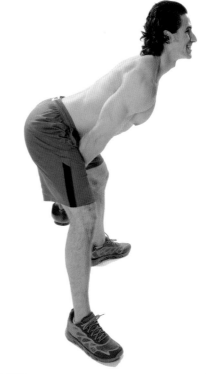

 Let your arms float up and bring the kettlebell to eye level.

4 Let the kettlebell fall naturally back to starting position.

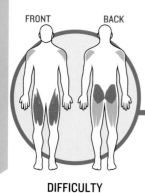

DIFFICULTY

Kettlebell Reverse Lunge Pass

Adding a kettlebell pass to the standard lunge requires focus and balance. This exercise works your quads, glutes, and hamstrings. You also get a workout for your core with the motion of passing the kettlebell between your legs.

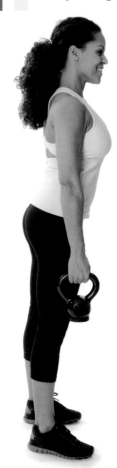

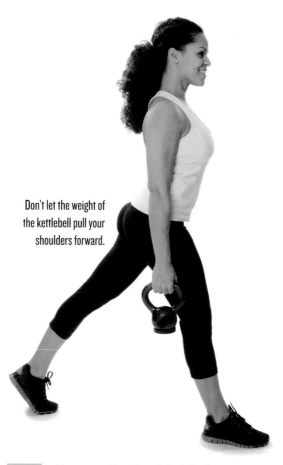

Don't let the weight of the kettlebell pull your shoulders forward.

1 Stand with your feet together. Hold the kettlebell in one hand down to your side.

2 Step one foot back behind you to prepare for the lunge.

Be Careful!

Don't let your knee extend past your toes during the lunge. Putting too much pressure on your knee joint can cause injury or long-term pain.

Keep in mind, you don't have to go into a full lunge if it causes you pain. Instead, you can go halfway down and work your way into doing the full lunge.

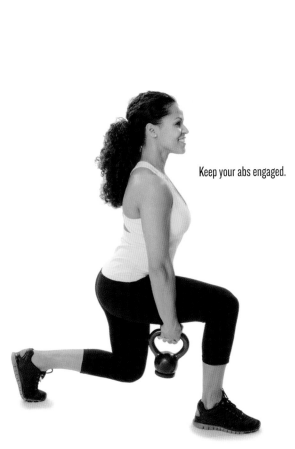

Keep your abs engaged.

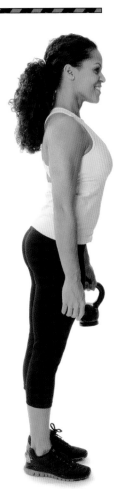

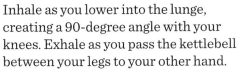

3 Inhale as you lower into the lunge, creating a 90-degree angle with your knees. Exhale as you pass the kettlebell between your legs to your other hand.

4 Inhale as you ascend back to starting position.

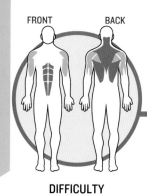

FRONT   BACK

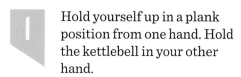

Kettlebell High Plank Row

This challenging version of the row requires the core strength to hold a plank with only one hand, because your other hand will be holding the kettlebell. This version of the plank works your abs, arms, and upper-body stability as you hold the plank, and the rhomboids and lats in your back as you do the row.

1 Hold yourself up in a plank position from one hand. Hold the kettlebell in your other hand.

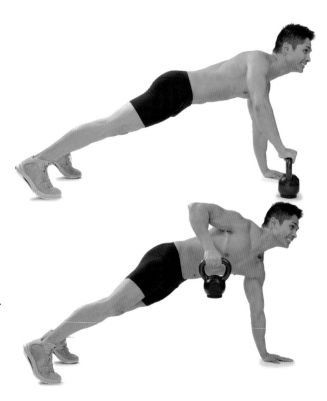

2 Inhale as you pull the kettlebell up to your side. At the top of the row, your elbow should be at a 90-degree angle.

If you feel your core begin to fail and your hips drop, you can perform this move from your knees. This allows you to keep proper form while doing the row.

3 Exhale as you lower the kettlebell back to the floor.

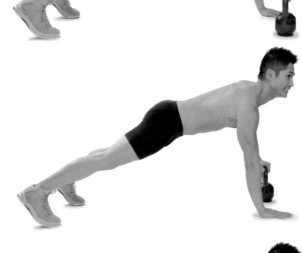

4 Transfer the kettlebell to your other hand.

5 Repeat the move, inhaling as you pull the kettlebell up to your side.

6 Exhale as you lower the kettlebell back to the floor.

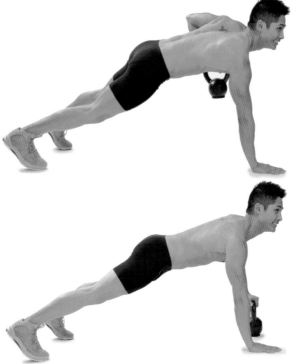

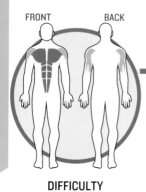

FRONT BACK

Kettlebell Sit-Up Press

This version of the sit-up incorporates the pecs and delts by adding a press at the top of the movement. This exercise also strengthens your abs and obliques and includes a balance challenge because of the addition of the kettlebell, which is held on one side of your body the entire time.

DIFFICULTY

1 Lie on the floor with your knees bent and your feet resting on the floor. Hold the kettlebell in one hand at your shoulder. Inhale as you stretch your abs.

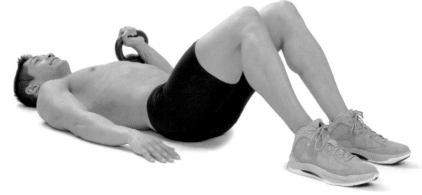

Rest the kettlebell on the back of your wrist for comfort.

2 Exhale as your lift your shoulders off the floor to contract your abs. Begin to press the kettlebell as you start the sit-up.

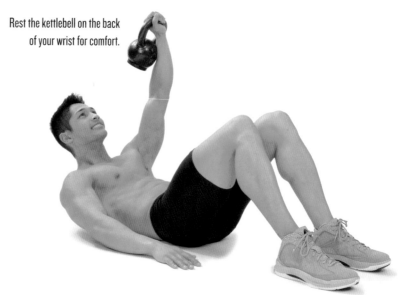

If the full sit-up seems a bit challenging, start with the crunch version of this exercise. You'll use the same core and upper-body muscles but with a smaller contraction in your midsection.

Keep your neck relaxed and focus on your abs crunching to pull you up.

Your hips and shoulders should face forward.

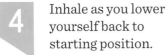 Continue pressing the kettlebell up as you reach the top of the sit-up.

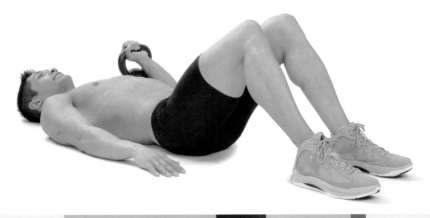

4 Inhale as you lower yourself back to starting position.

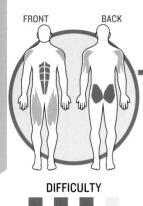

DIFFICULTY

Kettlebell Get-Up

The kettlebell get-up is a full-body exercise that takes you from lying flat on the floor to standing, all while you keep one arm straight up to the ceiling. The main focus is on your core stability; you must use your abdominals to ground your body as you stand up while holding the kettlebell straight up over your head. This exercise also works your legs, as their strength is needed when you stand up.

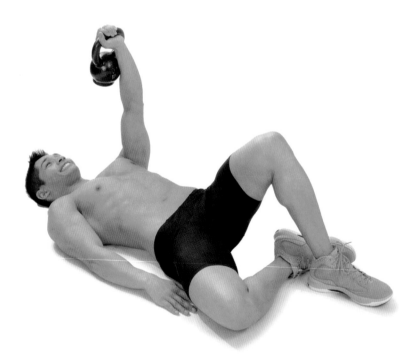

1 Lie flat on the floor with one arm stretched straight up toward the ceiling holding the kettlebell.

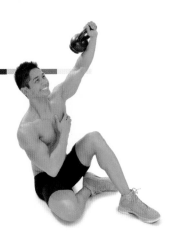

Variation
To progress the kettlebell get-up, take away your support arm. As this exercise is a total-body effort from start to finish, taking away the support will require even more core strength and focus to go from lying flat to standing up.

Keep your arm straight up for the entire move.

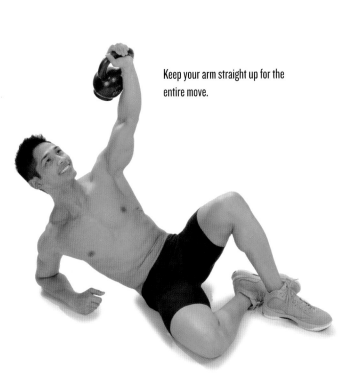

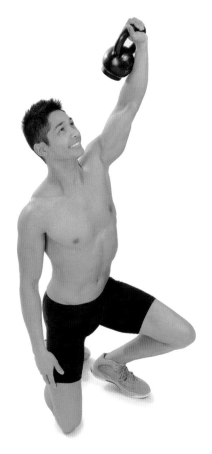

2 With the opposite arm acting as a support, lift your shoulders off the floor.

3 Tuck the leg on the same side as the support arm and begin to stand up with the opposite leg.

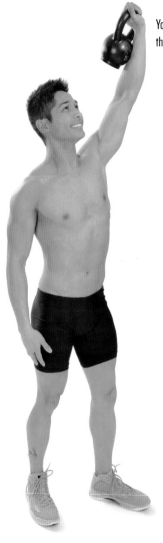

Your eyes should stay on the kettlebell.

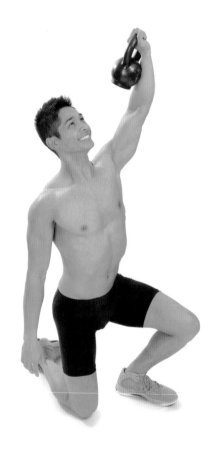

4 Stand all the way up with both feet flat while holding the kettlebell above your head.

5 Tuck your leg back under as your other leg lowers you back toward the floor.

6 As your hip reaches the floor, control your torso down with the support of your hand and elbow.

Continue to hold the kettlebell straight up in the air.

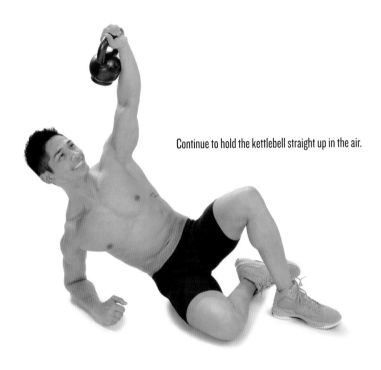

7 Lie back down to return to starting position.

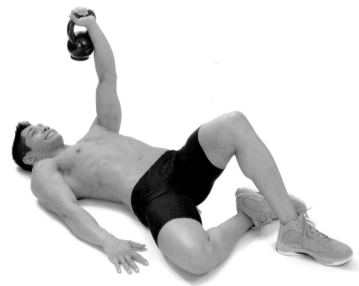

Suspension Bands

With suspension bands, you perform traditional exercises while your feet or hands are supported by these free-moving straps hanging from the ceiling—talk about difficult! You use a nice, steady tempo—which comes from the force of momentum—that conditions your energy systems to fire at higher, more efficient levels. Because your bodyweight is being used as resistance, suspension bands require your core muscles to always be actively engaged to support each and every rep. Also, suspension bands work stabilizing muscles that you may not have ever felt during traditional weight training.

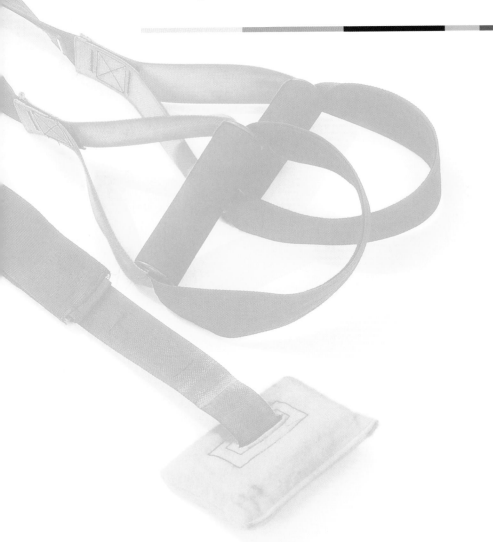

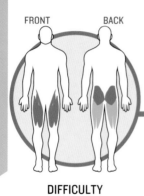

FRONT   BACK

DIFFICULTY

Suspension Band Squat and Single-Leg Squat

These versions of the squat and the single-leg squat allow you to have great form and proper technique through the support of the suspension bands. Both exercises use your bodyweight as resistance to target your gluteals (butt) and your hamstrings and quadriceps (legs).

Keep your head up and your eyes focused on the suspension bands.

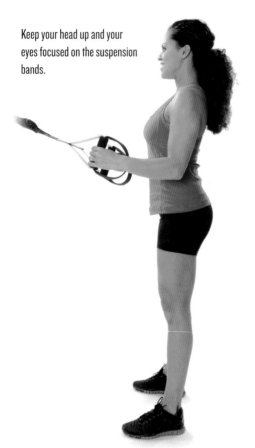

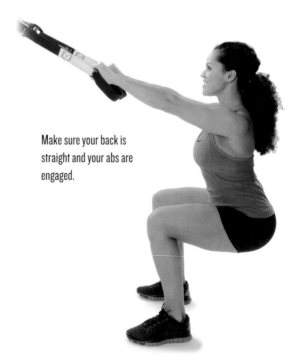

Make sure your back is straight and your abs are engaged.

1 Stand with your feet shoulder width apart. With the suspension bands in your hands, allow yourself to lean back.

2 Inhale as you lower into the squat, creating a 90-degree angle with your knees. Exhale as you rise back to starting position.

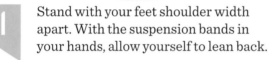

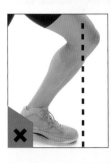
Even though you need a little help from your upper body to perform this move, your legs should do the majority of the work. Your arms will bend slightly during the squat, but use them more to help you maintain balance as you hold onto the suspension bands instead of as a way to pull yourself up out of the squat.

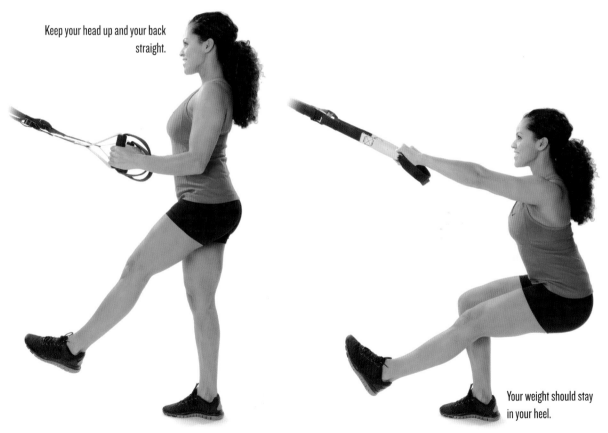

Keep your head up and your back straight.

Your weight should stay in your heel.

1 Balance on one foot with your opposite leg extended out in front of you. With the suspension bands in your hands, allow yourself to lean back.

2 Inhale as you lower into the squat, creating a 90-degree angle with your knee. Exhale as you rise back to starting position.

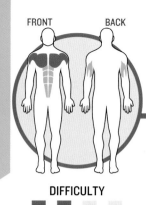

FRONT   BACK

DIFFICULTY

Suspension Band Chest Press and Chest Fly

With suspension bands, your bodyweight is used as resistance as you perform the chest press and chest fly. The suspension bands also provide a challenge to your core as you try to constantly stabilize your upper body. These exercises target your pecs, front delts, and triceps.

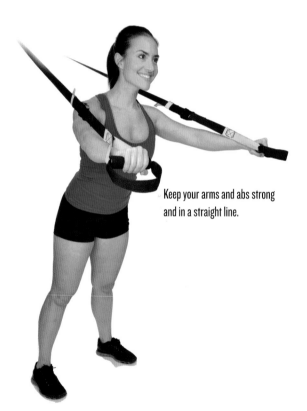

Your gaze should stay up and out to protect your spine.

Keep your arms and abs strong and in a straight line.

Your form should mimic a push-up.

1 Holding onto the handles with your palms facing down, lean away from the mounted suspension bands.

2 Inhale as you lower your body, creating a 90-degree angle with your elbows. Exhale as you ascend back to starting position.

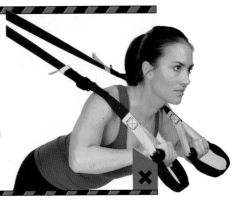

Be Careful!

Just as you do when performing the chest press and chest fly with dumbbells, be aware of your form. Placing too much pressure on your elbow joints by not using the suspension bands properly can cause pain and injury.

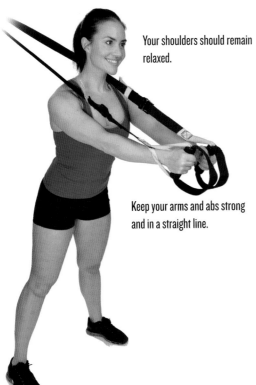

Your shoulders should remain relaxed.

Keep your arms and abs strong and in a straight line.

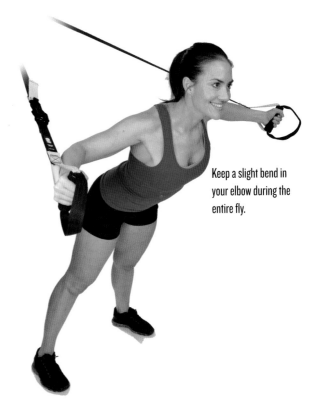

Keep a slight bend in your elbow during the entire fly.

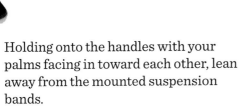

1 Holding onto the handles with your palms facing in toward each other, lean away from the mounted suspension bands.

2 Inhale as your arms open out to the sides to lower your body to stretch your pecs. Exhale as you ascend back to starting position.

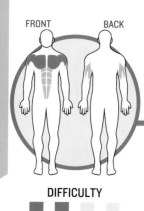

FRONT   BACK

DIFFICULTY

Suspension Band Row and Reverse Fly

Using suspension bands to perform the row and reverse fly requires constant stabilization in your upper body. In both exercises, your bodyweight acts as the resistance as your core keeps your body in a straight line. These exercises target your rhomboids, rear delts, and biceps.

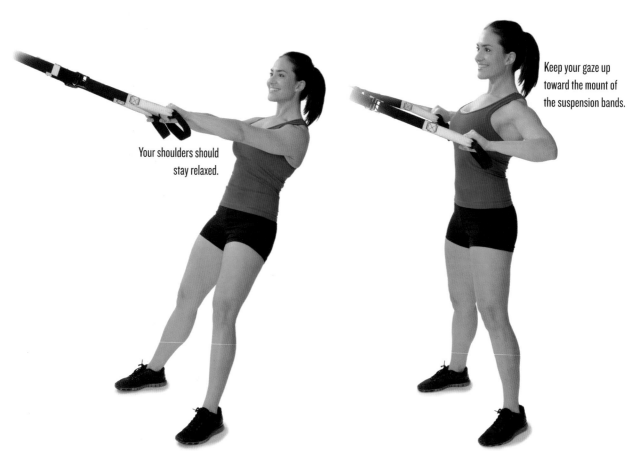

Your shoulders should stay relaxed.

Keep your gaze up toward the mount of the suspension bands.

1 Holding onto the handles with your palms facing down, lean away from the mounted suspension bands. Inhale as you engage your core and prepare to pull.

2 Exhale as you pull your body up into the row, creating a 90-degree angle with your elbows. Inhale as you descend back to starting position.

Be Careful!
As you do during the dumbbell versions of the row and reverse fly, watch out for your elbow joints. Also, start out at a slight angle and walk yourself down slowly to find the right starting position—don't make the angle of your body too drastic.

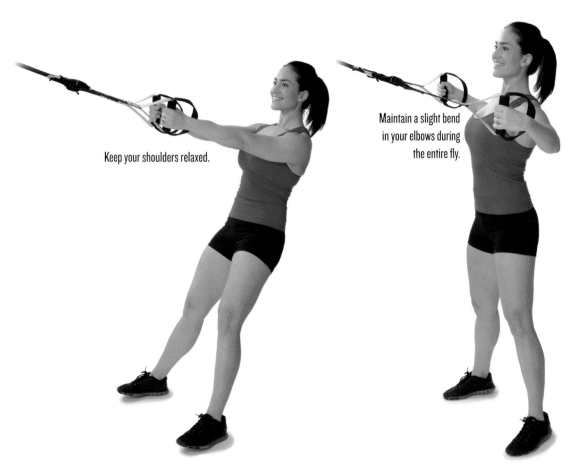

Keep your shoulders relaxed.

Maintain a slight bend in your elbows during the entire fly.

1 Holding onto the handles with your palms facing in toward each other, lean back from the mounted suspension bands. Inhale as you engage your core and prepare to fly.

2 Exhale as you open your arms out to your sides to contract your rhomboids. Inhale as you descend back to starting position.

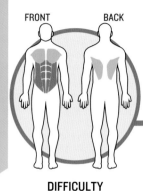

FRONT BACK

DIFFICULTY

Suspension Band Plank and Side Plank

Performing the plank and side plank from suspension bands increases the difficulty of these exercises. Because your feet aren't stable in the bands, your core muscles are challenged to hold your body up in a straight line.

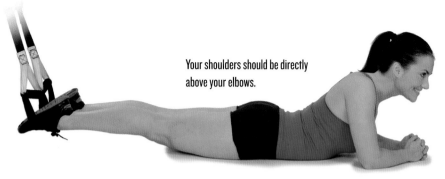

Your shoulders should be directly above your elbows.

1 Lie on your stomach with your feet in the straps of the suspension bands and your elbows resting on the floor.

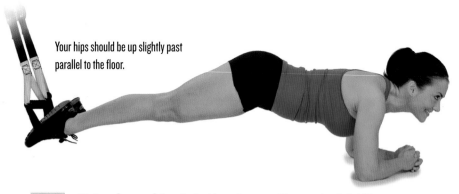

Your hips should be up slightly past parallel to the floor.

2 Extend your hips into the air, creating a straight line with your body. Breathe deeply while holding the plank.

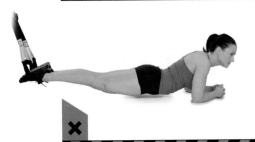

Be Careful!
Just like during a standard plank, pay attention to your form. Don't let your hips drop, or you'll potentially cause lower back pain and cause your abs to weaken and be unable to hold your body up in the plank.

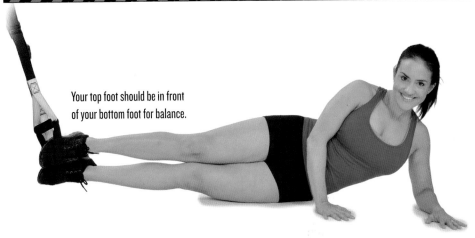

Your top foot should be in front of your bottom foot for balance.

1 Lie on your side with your feet in the straps of the suspension bands and one elbow resting on the floor.

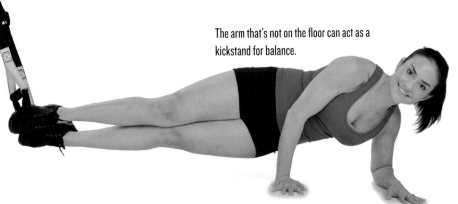

The arm that's not on the floor can act as a kickstand for balance.

2 Extend your hips up into the air, creating a straight line with your body. Breathe deeply while holding the plank.

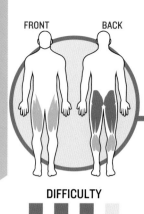

DIFFICULTY

Suspension Band Hamstring Roll

The suspension band hamstring roll is very similar to the bridge, but instead of starting in the bridge position, your feet move toward your body using your hamstrings. This exercise targets your glutes, hamstrings, and calves.

1 Lie on your back and place the heels of your feet in the suspension bands. Lift your hips up off the floor, creating a straight line with your body.

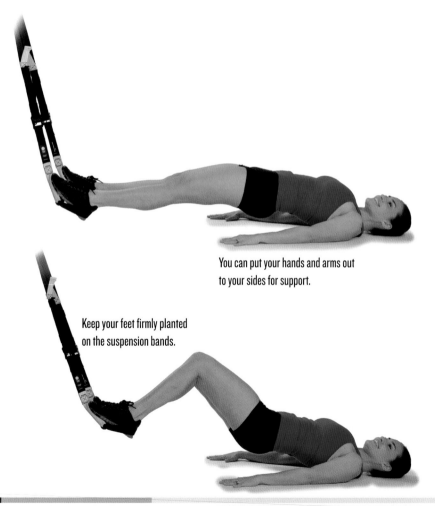

You can put your hands and arms out to your sides for support.

Keep your feet firmly planted on the suspension bands.

2 Exhale as you bring your feet in to contract your hamstrings.

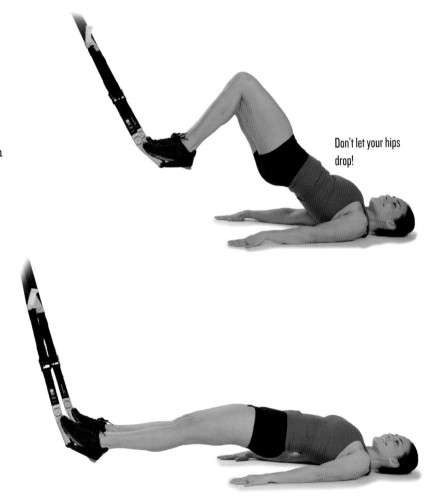

3 At the top of the roll, your knees, hips, and shoulders should be in a straight line.

Don't let your hips drop!

4 Inhale as you roll your heels back out to straight legs and return to starting position.

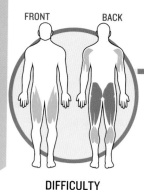

FRONT　　BACK

DIFFICULTY

Suspension Band Bridge

Using suspension bands can take a simple movement like the bridge and really up the difficulty. This exercise targets your glutes and hamstrings and even recruits muscles from your calves for stability.

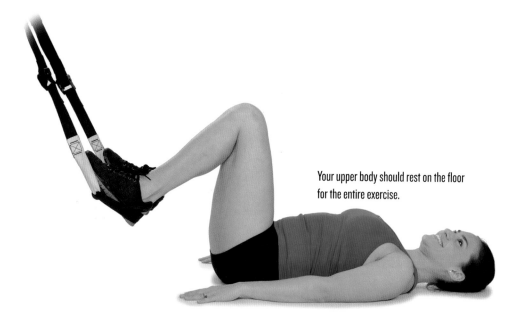

Your upper body should rest on the floor for the entire exercise.

Lie on your back with your knees bent and the heels of your feet in the suspension bands.

Be Careful!
Be sure to extend your hips all the way up and lower them all the way down to complete the bridge. Allowing your hips to drop midway without control may cause ankle or knee pain.

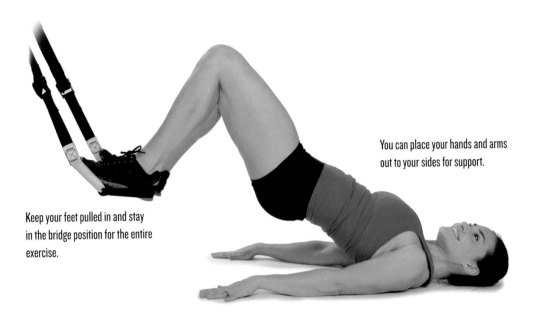

You can place your hands and arms
out to your sides for support.

Keep your feet pulled in and stay
in the bridge position for the entire
exercise.

2 Exhale as you press through your heels up into the
bridge. At the top of the bridge, your knees, hips, and
shoulders should be in a straight line.

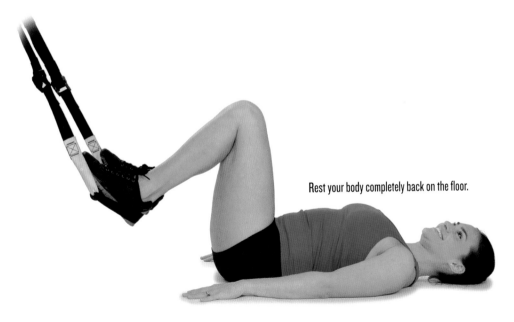

Rest your body completely back on the floor.

3 Inhale as you return back to starting position.

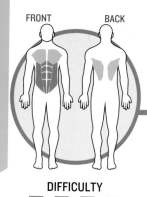

DIFFICULTY

Suspension Band Mountain Climber

In this powerful exercise, your abdominals are worked from beginning to end. The mountain climber engages your core with the push-up position and challenges your legs to stabilize as you climb using the suspended bands.

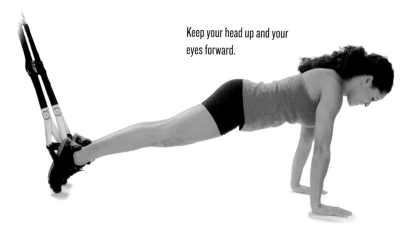

Keep your head up and your eyes forward.

1 With your feet suspended in the bands, hold yourself up in a plank from your hands. Inhale as you stretch and engage your abs.

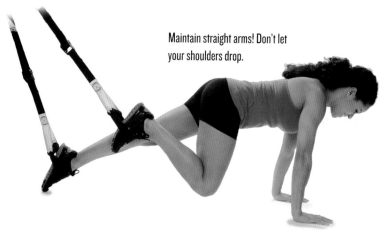

Maintain straight arms! Don't let your shoulders drop.

2 Exhale as you bring one knee forward to the center of your body in a climbing position.

3 After your climbing foot reaches the other back in starting position, repeat with the opposite knee.

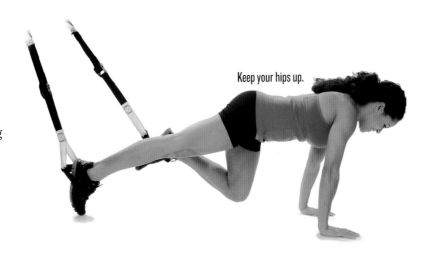

Keep your hips up.

4 Inhale as your return your knee to starting position.

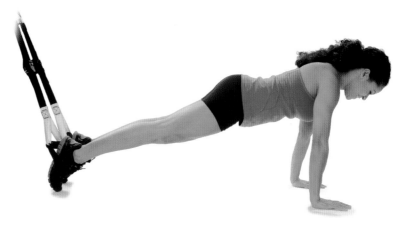

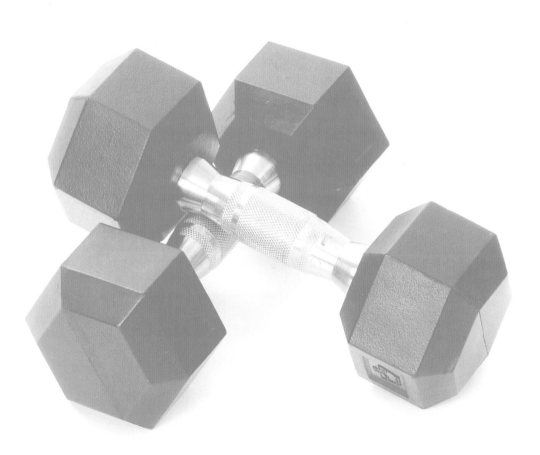

ROUTINES

In this part, I provide some weight-lifting routines you can follow, along with an example of each setup. Whether you only have a certain number of days a week to dedicate to going to the gym, a short time in which to work out, or a specific goal of fat loss or muscle building, I have made sure each routine takes into account all of your muscle groups.

When building a routine yourself, you should keep these things in mind:

1. **Muscle groups:** Involve every muscle group in your weekly routine.

2. **Intensity:** Design your routines so you push your body in a challenging way. Whether it's by going harder, slowing down and focusing on the tempo, or performing isometric exercises that use a static hold, you can vary the intensity of your routine.

3. **Time:** Pay attention to the time you spend on a routine, and recognize the fine line between too much and too little.

4. **Rest and recovery:** Give yourself plenty of rest between workouts.

5. **Progression:** Make sure you progress your routines once you've built your strength to a certain level, whether it's through moving up in weight, shorter breaks, more difficult movements, or supersets (pairing of exercises).

6. **Variation:** Choose a variety of exercises to challenge your muscles and avoid a plateau.

Two-Day Routine

Even if you only have two days a week to devote to weight training, you can still cover all your bases. This two-day split is an easy breakdown of upper and lower body. Try to spread out your lifting days evenly through the week (for example, Monday and Thursday) to allow your body to recover.

Day 1: Upper body (chest, back, shoulders, arms, and abs). Having only one day to cover all the muscles in your upper body may seem a little overwhelming, but you can manage it with the proper planning. Choose one main exercise for each muscle group and add from there—for example, a chest press (chest), a row (back), and a shoulder press (shoulders). If you feel the need to add arm- and ab-specific "simple exercises," that's fine, but simply be aware that your arms and abs will be involved in every exercise you do during day 1. Your arms will be worked during all the push-and-pull movements, while your abs will be pulled, crunched, and twisted during most of your weight lifting. You should be conscious of your core in particular because utilizing those muscles will help you strengthen your abs and lower back or core to the fullest.

Day 2: Lower body (quads, hamstrings, glutes, and calves). Because you have some of the largest muscles in your legs, you may find leg routines very draining. To help combat fatigue, always start with multi-joint movements that require both legs at the same time—for example, a squat. Starting with movement in the hip and knee joints will activate your muscles and also help you avoid injury when doing simpler leg exercises.

Day 1: Upper Body

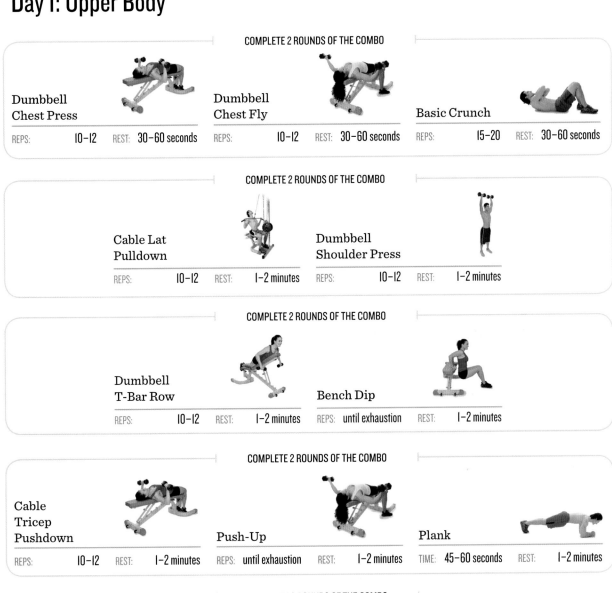

COMPLETE 2 ROUNDS OF THE COMBO

Dumbbell Chest Press
REPS: 10–12   REST: 30–60 seconds

Dumbbell Chest Fly
REPS: 10–12   REST: 30–60 seconds

Basic Crunch
REPS: 15–20   REST: 30–60 seconds

COMPLETE 2 ROUNDS OF THE COMBO

Cable Lat Pulldown
REPS: 10–12   REST: 1–2 minutes

Dumbbell Shoulder Press
REPS: 10–12   REST: 1–2 minutes

COMPLETE 2 ROUNDS OF THE COMBO

Dumbbell T-Bar Row
REPS: 10–12   REST: 1–2 minutes

Bench Dip
REPS: until exhaustion   REST: 1–2 minutes

COMPLETE 2 ROUNDS OF THE COMBO

Cable Tricep Pushdown
REPS: 10–12   REST: 1–2 minutes

Push-Up
REPS: until exhaustion   REST: 1–2 minutes

Plank
TIME: 45–60 seconds   REST: 1–2 minutes

COMPLETE 2 ROUNDS OF THE COMBO

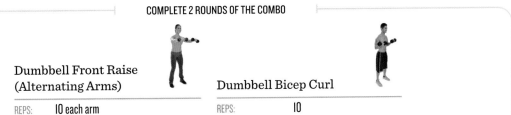

Dumbbell Front Raise (Alternating Arms)
REPS: 10 each arm

Dumbbell Bicep Curl
REPS: 10

Day 2: Lower Body

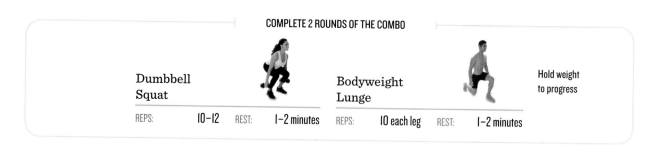

COMPLETE 2 ROUNDS OF THE COMBO

Dumbbell Squat

REPS: 10–12   REST: 1–2 minutes

Bodyweight Lunge

REPS: 10 each leg   REST: 1–2 minutes

Hold weight to progress

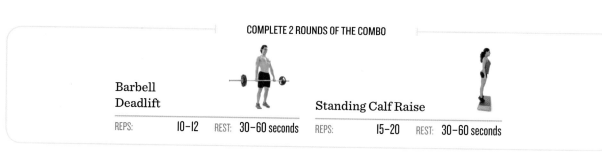

COMPLETE 2 ROUNDS OF THE COMBO

Barbell Deadlift

REPS: 10–12   REST: 30–60 seconds

Standing Calf Raise

REPS: 15–20   REST: 30–60 seconds

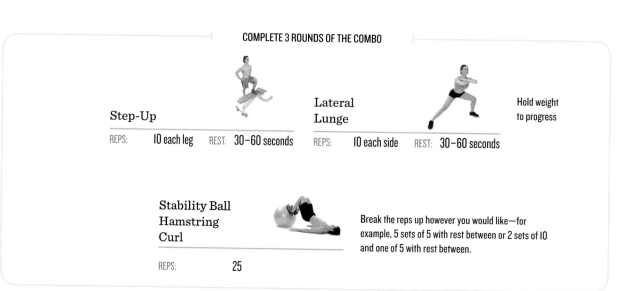

COMPLETE 3 ROUNDS OF THE COMBO

Step-Up

REPS: 10 each leg   REST: 30–60 seconds

Lateral Lunge

REPS: 10 each side   REST: 30–60 seconds

Hold weight to progress

Stability Ball Hamstring Curl

REPS: 25

Break the reps up however you would like—for example, 5 sets of 5 with rest between or 2 sets of 10 and one of 5 with rest between.

Three-Day Routine

Having more days in which to divide up your lifts can be beneficial. With a three-day split, you can break up the upper-body muscles into two days. One way you can structure your routine is to simply have a workout day followed by a rest day. Another way you can do this routine is to build in a rest day or days for the weekend and then repeat your series again as Monday comes around—for example, a Monday-Wednesday-Friday schedule.

Day 1: Chest and back. These are like the yin and yang of your upper body. When you work your chest and back, you push and pull with opposing muscles groups—for example, in a chest press, the chest muscles work as the agonists, pulling one way, while the back muscles work as the antagonists, pulling the other way.

Day 2: Legs and abs. Combining legs and abs in a routine is quite easy because big lower-body exercises require a strong core to be performed properly. This is especially important to keep in mind when both legs and abs are trained together, as your hip flexors will be activated in all of your leg exercises.

Day 3: Shoulders and arms. Training your arms with your shoulders is very complementary, because your biceps and triceps are involved in shoulder exercises. For example, your triceps assist during a shoulder press and your biceps help pull during an upright row. And as you exhaust your arms, you'll begin to rely more on your delts during the lateral and front raises, which works your shoulders. Keep in mind that both your arms and shoulders are known to be helpers for many other muscle groups, so it's important to rest and recover after this day!

Day I: Chest and Back

Pull-Up

REPS: until exhaustion   REST: 30–60 seconds

Seated Cable Low Row

REPS: 10   REST: 30–60 seconds

Dumbbell Chest Press

REPS: 10–12   REST: 30–60 seconds

Push-Up

REPS: until exhaustion   REST: 30–60 seconds

Dumbbell Pullover

REPS: 10   REST: 30–60 seconds

Dumbbell Chest Fly

REPS: 10–12   REST: 30–60 seconds

Dumbbell One-Arm Row

REPS: 10–12   REST: 30–60 seconds

Decline Push-Up

REPS: until exhaustion   REST: 30–60 seconds

Day 2: Legs and Abs

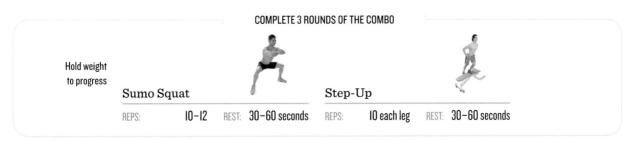

COMPLETE 3 ROUNDS OF THE COMBO

Hold weight
to progress

Sumo Squat

REPS: 10-12   REST: 30-60 seconds

Step-Up

REPS: 10 each leg   REST: 30-60 seconds

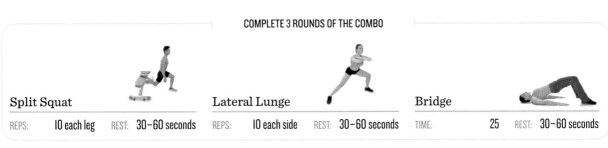

COMPLETE 3 ROUNDS OF THE COMBO

**Dumbbell
Straight-Leg
Deadlift**

REPS: 10-12   REST: 30-60 seconds

Standing Calf Raise

REPS: until exhaustion   REST: 30-60 seconds

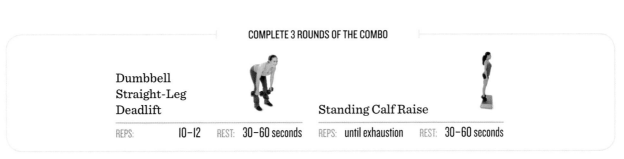

COMPLETE 3 ROUNDS OF THE COMBO

Split Squat

REPS: 10 each leg   REST: 30-60 seconds

Lateral Lunge

REPS: 10 each side   REST: 30-60 seconds

Bridge

TIME: 25   REST: 30-60 seconds

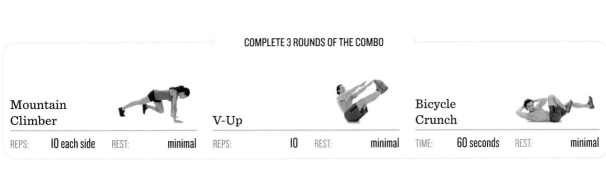

COMPLETE 3 ROUNDS OF THE COMBO

**Mountain
Climber**

REPS: 10 each side   REST: minimal

V-Up

REPS: 10   REST: minimal

**Bicycle
Crunch**

TIME: 60 seconds   REST: minimal

Day 3: Shoulders and Arms

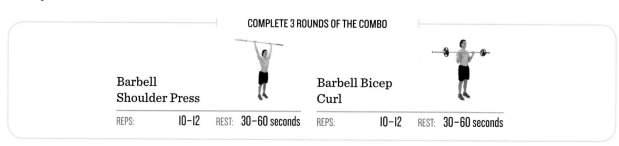

COMPLETE 3 ROUNDS OF THE COMBO

Barbell
Shoulder Press

REPS: 10–12   REST: 30–60 seconds

Barbell Bicep
Curl

REPS: 10–12   REST: 30–60 seconds

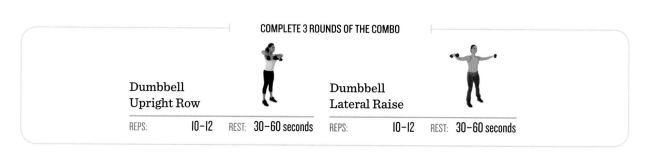

COMPLETE 3 ROUNDS OF THE COMBO

Dumbbell
Upright Row

REPS: 10–12   REST: 30–60 seconds

Dumbbell
Lateral Raise

REPS: 10–12   REST: 30–60 seconds

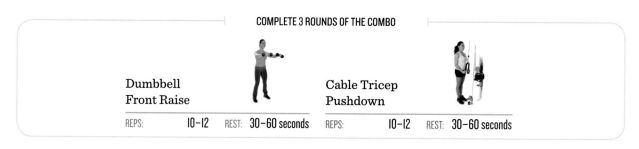

COMPLETE 3 ROUNDS OF THE COMBO

Dumbbell
Front Raise

REPS: 10–12   REST: 30–60 seconds

Cable Tricep
Pushdown

REPS: 10–12   REST: 30–60 seconds

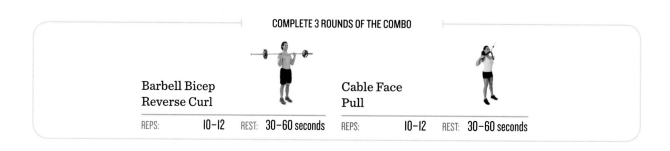

COMPLETE 3 ROUNDS OF THE COMBO

Barbell Bicep
Reverse Curl

REPS: 10–12   REST: 30–60 seconds

Cable Face
Pull

REPS: 10–12   REST: 30–60 seconds

Four-Day Routine

A four-day routine lets you divide up your lifts even more, with more specific muscle targets each day. However, don't get carried away and start moving toward an everyday lifting schedule—otherwise, your muscles won't be able to recover properly and you'll get burnt out fast. In the case of a four-day routine, I recommend keeping a day of rest between workouts if you can.

Day 1: Chest and triceps. These muscle groups pair well in a routine because you use the triceps in your arms to do the chest exercises. For example, in all the chest press type of exercises, your triceps are always the secondary muscles used, because as your arms straighten out at the top of the press, your triceps are fully extended to help assist the completion of the move.

Day 2: Legs. Your legs are powerfully built with big muscles. They can do some major work, and require a lot of energy. Focusing on your legs as the single muscle trained is very smart because there are so many large muscles to be broken down. You will use hip flexion and extension to target the glutes, hamstrings, and quads to develop a strong and functional lower body.

Day 3: Back and biceps. As the chest and triceps are during day 1, the back and biceps are paired together because they work hand-in-hand—in this case, during the vertical or horizontal pulling movements of cable exercises. When you're doing a vertical or horizontal pull to work your back muscles, the biceps in your arms are going to be used to complete the move. Your biceps are also utilized more and more as the angle in your elbow decreases. So during a pull-up, for example, you'll pull more from your lats at the beginning, but your biceps will contract more as you reach the top.

Day 4: Shoulders and abs. At the end of the week, you may look forward to an easier lifting routine. Because shoulders and abs are smaller muscles that require less energy and tend to recover quickly, you can end your week with exercises focusing on them.

Day I: Chest and Triceps

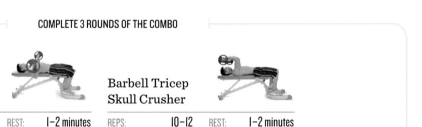

COMPLETE 3 ROUNDS OF THE COMBO

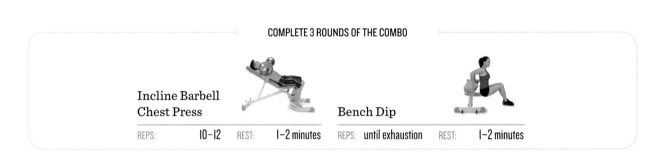

Barbell Chest Press

REPS: 10–12   REST: 1–2 minutes

Barbell Tricep Skull Crusher

REPS: 10–12   REST: 1–2 minutes

COMPLETE 3 ROUNDS OF THE COMBO

Incline Barbell Chest Press

REPS: 10–12   REST: 1–2 minutes

Bench Dip

REPS: until exhaustion   REST: 1–2 minutes

COMPLETE 3 ROUNDS OF THE COMBO

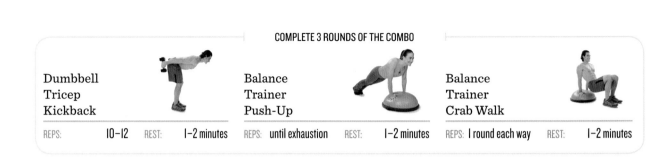

Dumbbell Tricep Kickback

REPS: 10–12   REST: 1–2 minutes

Balance Trainer Push-Up

REPS: until exhaustion   REST: 1–2 minutes

Balance Trainer Crab Walk

REPS: 1 round each way   REST: 1–2 minutes

Day 2: Legs

COMPLETE 3 ROUNDS OF THE COMBO

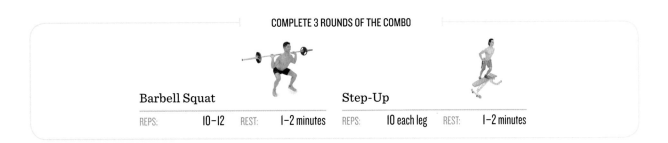

Barbell Squat

REPS: 10–12   REST: 1–2 minutes

Step-Up

REPS: 10 each leg   REST: 1–2 minutes

COMPLETE 3 ROUNDS OF THE COMBO

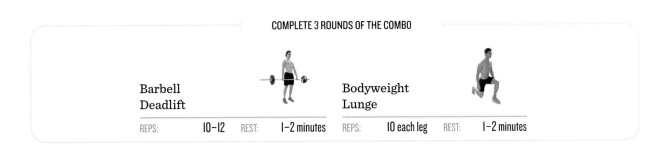

Barbell Deadlift

REPS: 10–12   REST: 1–2 minutes

Bodyweight Lunge

REPS: 10 each leg   REST: 1–2 minutes

COMPLETE 3 ROUNDS OF THE COMBO

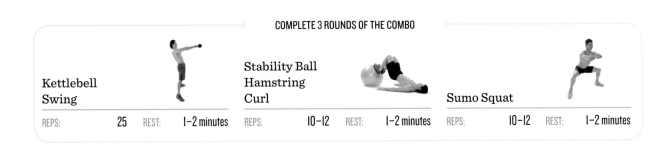

Kettlebell Swing

REPS: 25   REST: 1–2 minutes

Stability Ball Hamstring Curl

REPS: 10–12   REST: 1–2 minutes

Sumo Squat

REPS: 10–12   REST: 1–2 minutes

Day 3: Back and Biceps

COMPLETE 3 ROUNDS OF THE COMBO

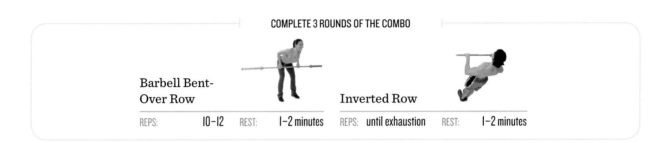

Barbell Bent-Over Row

REPS: 10-12   REST: 1-2 minutes

Inverted Row

REPS: until exhaustion   REST: 1-2 minutes

COMPLETE 3 ROUNDS OF THE COMBO

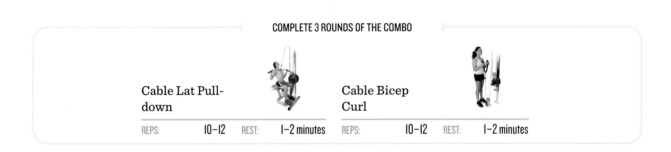

Cable Lat Pull-down

REPS: 10-12   REST: 1-2 minutes

Cable Bicep Curl

REPS: 10-12   REST: 1-2 minutes

COMPLETE 3 ROUNDS OF THE COMBO

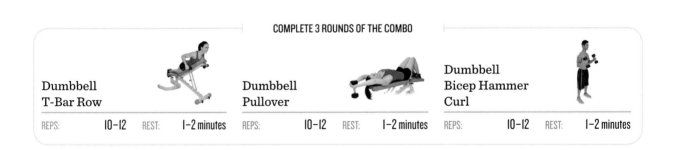

Dumbbell T-Bar Row

REPS: 10-12   REST: 1-2 minutes

Dumbbell Pullover

REPS: 10-12   REST: 1-2 minutes

Dumbbell Bicep Hammer Curl

REPS: 10-12   REST: 1-2 minutes

Day 4: Shoulders and Abs

COMPLETE 3 ROUNDS OF THE COMBO

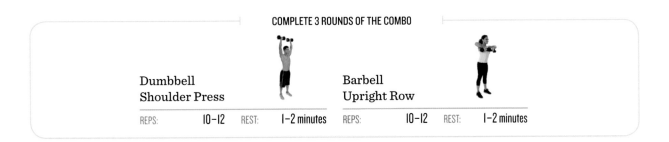

Dumbbell
Shoulder Press

REPS: 10–12 REST: 1–2 minutes

Barbell
Upright Row

REPS: 10–12 REST: 1–2 minutes

COMPLETE 3 ROUNDS OF THE COMBO

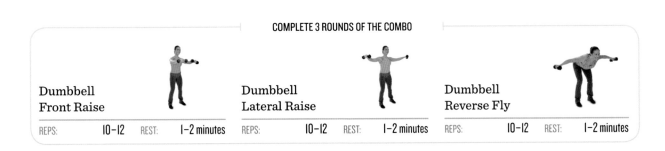

Dumbbell
Front Raise

REPS: 10–12 REST: 1–2 minutes

Dumbbell
Lateral Raise

REPS: 10–12 REST: 1–2 minutes

Dumbbell
Reverse Fly

REPS: 10–12 REST: 1–2 minutes

COMPLETE 3 ROUNDS OF THE COMBO

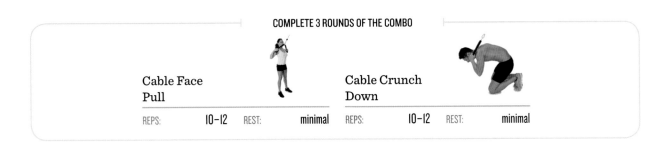

Cable Face
Pull

REPS: 10–12 REST: minimal

Cable Crunch
Down

REPS: 10–12 REST: minimal

Full Body in 15 Routine

Sometimes the responsibilities of housework, your job, and your family don't leave you a whole lot of spare time to work out. If you're crunched for time, try one of the following full-body routines—you only need 15 minutes! The best part is that all of these routines can be done in your home with a set of dumbbells—15- to 20-pound dumbbells for men and 5- to 10-pound dumbbells for women to start with. You can move up in weight as you need to progress.

When building a 15-minute routine yourself, a nice place to start is legs, with exercises such as bodyweight squats and lunges. You can then move on to your upper body and incorporate your core using any version of the push-ups. You only need your bodyweight to perform some of the most effective exercises, so keep that in mind when designing your routine.

Booty Lift

COMPLETE AS MANY ROUNDS OF THE COMBO AS YOU CAN IN 15 MINUTES

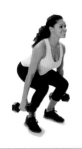

Dumbbell Squat

REPS: 10   REST: none

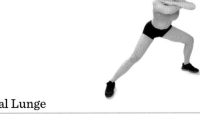

Lateral Lunge

REPS: 10 each side   REST: none

Mountain Climber

REPS: 15 each side   REST: none

Bridge

REPS: 25   REST: none

Popeye Pump

COMPLETE 2 ROUNDS OF THE ENTIRE ROUTINE

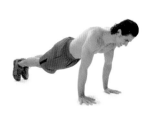

Push-Up

REPS: 10   REST: **30-60 seconds**

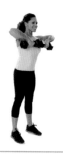

Bodyweight Lunge

REPS: 10   REST: **30-60 seconds**

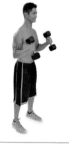

Dumbbell Bicep Hammer Curl

REPS: 10   REST: **30-60 seconds**

Dumbbell Upright Row

REPS: 10   REST: **30-60 seconds**

Push-Up

REPS: 10   REST: **30-60 seconds**

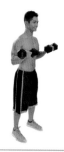

Dumbbell Bicep Curl

REPS: 15   REST: **30-60 seconds**

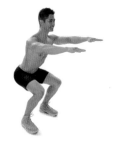

Bodyweight Squat

REPS: 15   REST: **30-60 seconds**

Dumbbell Bent-Over Row

REPS: 15   REST: **30-60 seconds**

Energy Boost and Fat Burn

COMPLETE AS MANY ROUNDS OF THE COMBO AS YOU CAN IN 15 MINUTES

Sumo Squat with Dumbbell Shoulder Press at Top

| REPS: | 10 | REST: | none |

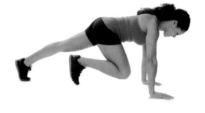

Dumbbell Lateral Raise

| REPS: | 10 | REST: | none |

Mountain Climber

| REPS: | 15 each side | REST: | none |

Push-Up

| REPS: | until exhaustion | REST: | none |

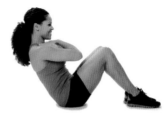

Sit-Up

| REPS: | 10 | REST: | none |

Lengthen and Stretch

COMPLETE 2 ROUNDS OF THE ENTIRE ROUTINE

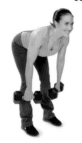

**Dumbbell
Straight-Leg
Deadlift**

REPS: 10   REST: 30-60 seconds

**Get-Up (using
a kettlebell or a
dumbbell)**

REPS: 5 each side   REST: 30-60 seconds

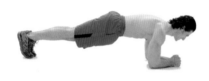

Plank

TIME: 45–60 seconds   REST: 30-60 seconds

**Dumbbell
Tricep
Kickback**

REPS: 10   REST: 30-60 seconds

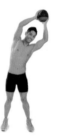

**Worship
Stretch**

REPS: 10 each side   REST: 30-60 seconds

**Dumbbell
Shoulder Press**

REPS: 10   REST: 30-60 seconds

Weight Loss Routine

When weight loss is the goal, it's important to keep your workouts moving quickly, with fast-paced exercises. You should also do higher reps, because your goal is to condition the muscle you have instead of growing new muscle. To accomplish this, choose weights with which you can complete 12 to 15 reps—nothing too heavy. This full-body routine should give you a toned and tight feeling, with little soreness afterward. Rest three to five days before repeating the routine.

When designing a weight loss routine yourself, have a few staple exercises you know you enjoy and give you a great sweat, like kettlebell swings, walking lunges, and mountain climbers.

To progress the squat and shoulder press, combine them so that you shoulder press at the top of your squat.

Dumbbell Squat

REPS: 12-15   REST: minimal

Dumbbell Shoulder Press

REPS: 12-15   REST: minimal

Stability Ball Hamstring Curl

REPS: 12-15   REST: minimal

Bicycle Crunch

TIME: 60 seconds   REST: minimal

COMPLETE 3 ROUNDS OF THE COMBO

Dumbbell Chest Press

REPS: until exhaustion   REST: minimal

Reverse Crunch

REPS: 15-20   REST: minimal

Kettlebell Swing

REPS: 15-20   REST: minimal

Kettlebell Reverse Lunge Pass

REPS: 10 each side   REST: minimal

COMPLETE 3 ROUNDS OF THE COMBO

Dumbbell Bent-Over Row

REPS: 12-15   REST: minimal

Suspension Band Mountain Climber

REPS: 15 each leg   REST: minimal

Dumbbell Tricep Kickback

REPS: 12-15   REST: minimal

Muscle Gain Routine

For this full-body routine, you're looking to break down the muscles so they can grow. Therefore, it's heavier and slower moving than other routines, with more days of rest in between. You'll be very sore afterward, so make sure you give yourself five to eight days of rest. If you're still sore after this time, add on another day of rest.

When designing your own lifting routine for gaining muscle size and strength, always start out by choosing at least one exercise for each major muscle group. If you spend time doing extra movements for the same muscle group, you'll most likely tire out, which will keep you from completing the other muscle groups. Also, if you exhaust your arms during a major-movement exercise, like a pull-up or bodyweight dip, your arms will need more time to rest before moving on to the next exercise; this can affect the performance of the rest of your workout. Choose carefully, and allow yourself to take good, long breaks.

COMPLETE 3 ROUNDS OF THE COMBO

Pull-Up

REPS: until exhaustion   REST: 1–2 minutes

Barbell Squat

REPS: 6–8   REST: 1–2 minutes

COMPLETE 3 ROUNDS OF THE COMBO

Dumbbell Deadlift

REPS: 6–8   REST: 1–2 minutes

Dumbbell Bicep Hammer Curl

REPS: 6–8   REST: 1–2 minutes

You can alternate these two exercises with every rep to make them one big movement—for example, you can perform a deadlift with a curl at the top.

COMPLETE 3 ROUNDS OF THE COMBO

Incline Dumbbell Chest Press

REPS: 6–8   REST: 1–2 minutes

COMPLETE 3 ROUNDS OF THE COMBO

Barbell Tricep Skull Crusher

REPS: 6–8   REST: 1–2 minutes

Bodyweight Dip

REPS: until exhaustion   REST: 1–2 minutes

Hanging Leg Lift

REPS: 8–10   REST: 1–2 minutes